STUDENT UNIT GUIDE

NEW EDITION

AQA AS Biology Unit 1
Biology and Disease

Steve Potter and Martin Rowland

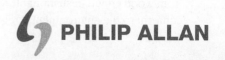

PHILIP ALLAN

Philip Allan Updates, an imprint of Hodder Education, an Hachette UK company, Market Place, Deddington, Oxfordshire OX15 0SE

Orders
Bookpoint Ltd, 130 Milton Park, Abingdon, Oxfordshire, OX14 4SB
tel: 01235 827827
fax: 01235 400401
e-mail: education@bookpoint.co.uk
Lines are open 9.00 a.m.–5.00 p.m., Monday to Saturday, with a 24-hour message answering service.
You can also order through the Philip Allan Updates website: www.philipallan.co.uk

ISBN 978-1-4441-5286-9

First printed 2011
Impression number 5 4 3
Year 2015 2014 2013

Cover photo: fusebulb/Fotolia

Printed in Dubai

Hachette UK's policy is to use papers that are natural, renewable and recyclable products and made from wood grown in sustainable forests. The logging and manufacturing processes are expected to conform to the environmental regulations of the country of origin.

P01938

Contents

Getting the most from this book 4

About this book 5

Content Guidance

How disease is caused 8

The molecules in our food 12

The structure and functioning of the digestive system 20

Cell structure and the absorption of the products of digestion 27

The lungs, breathing and gas exchange 39

The structure and functioning of the heart 47

The body's reaction to infection 53

Questions & Answers

Q1 Heart disease and risk factors 59

Q2 The molecules in our food 61

Q3 The structure and functioning of the digestive system 63

Q4 The nature and action of enzymes 65

Q5 Cell structure and the absorption of the products of digestion (I) 68

Q6 Cell structure and the absorption of the products of digestion (II) 70

Q7 The lungs, breathing and gas exchange 74

Q8 The structure and functioning of the heart 76

Q9 Smoking and respiratory disease 79

Q10 Monoclonal antibodies 82

Knowledge check answers 84

Index 85

Getting the most from this book

Examiner tips

Advice from the examiner on key points in the text to help you learn and recall unit content, avoid pitfalls, and polish your exam technique in order to boost your grade.

Knowledge check

Rapid-fire questions throughout the Content Guidance section to check your understanding.

Knowledge check answers

1 Turn to the back of the book for the Knowledge check answers.

Summary

Summaries

- Each core topic is rounded off by a bullet-list summary for quick-check reference of what you need to know.

Questions & Answers

Exam-style questions

Examiner comments on the questions
Tips on what you need to do to gain full marks, indicated by the icon ⓔ.

Sample student answers
Practise the questions, then look at the student answers that follow each set of questions.

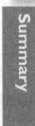

Examiner commentary on sample student answers
Find out how many marks each answer would be awarded in the exam and then read the examiner comments (preceded by the icon ⓔ) following each student answer. Annotations that link back to points made in the student answers show exactly how and where marks are gained or lost.

AQA AS Biology

About this book

This guide will help you to prepare for **BIOL1**, the examination for **Unit 1: Biology and Disease** of the AQA A-level Biology specification. Although BIOL1 forms part of the AS assessment, your understanding of some of the principles in Unit 1 may be re-examined in A2 unit tests.

The **Content Guidance** section covers all the facts you need to know and concepts you need to understand for BIOL1. In each topic, the concepts are presented first. It is a good idea to get your mind around these key ideas before you try to learn all the associated facts. The Content Guidance also includes examiner tips and knowledge checks to help you prepare for BIOL1.

The **Question and Answer** section shows you the sorts of questions you can expect in the unit test. It would be impossible to give examples of every kind of question in one book, but these should give you a flavour of what to expect. Each question has been attempted by two students, Student A and Student B. Their answers, along with the examiner's comments, should help you to see what you need to do to score a good mark — and how you can easily *not* score a mark even though you probably understand the biology.

What can I assume about this book?

You can assume that:
- the basic facts you need to know and understand are stated explicitly
- the major concepts you need to understand are explained clearly
- the questions at the end of the guide are similar in style to those that will appear in the BIOL1 unit test
- some of the questions test aspects of *How Science Works*
- the answers supplied are the answers of AS students
- the standard of the marking is broadly equivalent to that which will be applied to your answers

So how should I use this book?

The guide lends itself to a number of uses throughout your course — it is not *just* a revision aid. You could:
- use it to check that your notes cover the material required by the specification
- use it to identify your strengths and weaknesses
- use it as a reference for homework and internal tests
- use it during your revision to prepare 'bite-sized' chunks of related material, rather than being faced with a file full of notes

You could use the Question and Answer section to:
- identify the terms used by examiners and show what they expect of you
- familiarise yourself with the style of questions you can expect
- identify the ways in which students gain, or fail to gain, marks

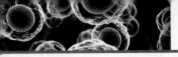

Develop *your* examination strategy

Just as reading the *Highway Code* alone will not help you to pass your driving test, this guide cannot help to make you a good examination candidate unless you develop and maintain all the skills that examiners will test in BIOL1. You also need to be aware of the type of questions examiners ask and where to find them in the unit test. You can then develop your own personal examination strategy. But, be warned, this is a highly personal and long-term process; you cannot do it a few days before the unit test.

Things you *must* do

- Clearly, you must know some biology. If you don't, you cannot expect to get a good grade. This guide provides a succinct summary of the biology you must know.
- Be aware of the skills that examiners *must* test in BIOL1. These are called assessment objectives and are described in the AQA Biology specification.
- Understand the weighting of the assessment objectives that will be used in BIOL1. Examiners have designed BIOL1 with the approximate balance of marks shown in the table.

Assessment objective	Brief summary	Marks in BIOL1
AO1	Knowledge and understanding	26
AO2	Application of knowledge and understanding	26
AO3	*How Science Works*	8

- Use past questions and other exercises to develop all the skills that examiners must test. Once you have developed them all, keep practising to maintain them.
- Understand where in BIOL1 different types of questions occur. For example, the final question will always be worth 10 marks and will test AO1 by requiring you to write extended prose. If that is the skill in which you feel most comfortable, and many AS students do, why not attempt this question first?

Content Guidance

This section is a guide to the content of **Unit 1: Biology and Disease**. In addition to the following features, each of the sections headed 'The biological basis of related disease' describes disease(s) that affect the functioning of the system just covered.

Key concepts you must understand

Whereas you can learn facts, these are ideas or concepts that may form the basis of models that we use to explain aspects of biology. You can know the words that describe concepts like osmosis, but you will not be able to use this information unless you really understand what is going on.

Key facts you must know and understand

These are exactly what you might think: a summary of the basic knowledge that you must be able to recall and show that you understand. The knowledge has been broken down into a number of small facts that you must learn. This means that the list of 'Key facts' for some topics is quite long. However, this approach makes quite clear *everything* you need to know about the topic.

Summary

This part describes the skills you should be able to demonstrate after studying the relevant topic. These include the skills associated with the assessment objectives that examiners will ask you to demonstrate in the BIOL1 unit test.

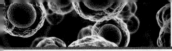

Content Guidance

How disease is caused

Key concepts you must understand

Disease is 'a condition with a specific cause in which part or all of an organism is made to function in an abnormal or less efficient manner'.

Disease results from:

- pathogenic organisms (bacteria, viruses, fungi and protoctistans). These diseases are called **infectious diseases**.
- a person's lifestyle and working conditions. Examples include many cancers, some forms of heart disease and fibrosis.
- degenerative processes. These are often the result of ageing and include arthritis and atherosclerosis.
- inherited gene mutations. Examples include haemophilia and phenylketonuria.
- nutrient deficiency. Examples include scurvy (caused by a lack of vitamin C in the diet) and kwashiorkor (caused by a lack of protein in the diet).

Pre-existing knowledge

Much of the evidence linking the various risk factors to coronary heart disease and to some cancers is **epidemiological** and **correlational**. Epidemiologists study the incidence of different diseases in different groups of people. When they find a high correlation between a particular group of people (e.g. smokers) and disease (e.g. lung cancer), they can *suggest*, but not definitely *prove*, cause and effect. This suggestion can then lead to scientific investigations into cause and effect.

Key facts you must know and understand

Infectious diseases

Infection can take place wherever there is an *interface* between the body and the environment. Figure 1 shows the main interfaces, together with the ways in which infection is resisted.

Organisms that cause disease are called **pathogens**. The process by which a pathogen enters and becomes established in an organism to cause disease is called **infection**.

Most infectious diseases are caused by bacteria, viruses or fungi. The table below describes how each type of pathogen causes disease.

examiner tip

Don't refer to the disease itself as an infection. Disease is a condition; infection is a process.

examiner tip

The specification requires you to name only two interfaces of the body — the digestive system and the respiratory system.

examiner tip

You will not be rewarded for using the term 'germs' in a unit test. Instead, you must use appropriately the terms pathogens, bacteria, viruses or fungi.

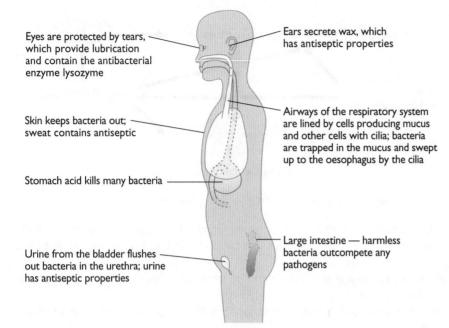

Eyes are protected by tears, which provide lubrication and contain the antibacterial enzyme lysozyme

Ears secrete wax, which has antiseptic properties

Skin keeps bacteria out; sweat contains antiseptic

Airways of the respiratory system are lined by cells producing mucus and other cells with cilia; bacteria are trapped in the mucus and swept up to the oesophagus by the cilia

Stomach acid kills many bacteria

Urine from the bladder flushes out bacteria in the urethra; urine has antiseptic properties

Large intestine — harmless bacteria outcompete any pathogens

Figure 1 The body's interfaces have mechanisms that resist infection

Type of microorganism	How the microorganism causes disease	Example of disease caused
Bacterium	Bacteria release toxins as they multiply. These toxins affect cells in the region of the infection and sometimes also in other regions of the body. Bacterial diseases can be treated with antibiotics because each bacterium is a cell with its own 'metabolic pathways' and is capable of cell division.	Pulmonary tuberculosis (TB); pneumonia; cholera
Virus	Viruses enter living cells and disrupt them. The genetic material of the virus becomes incorporated into that of the cell and instructs the cell to produce more viruses. Diseases caused by viruses cannot be treated with antibiotics because viruses do not have their own metabolic pathways.	Influenza (flu); AIDS; measles; common cold
Fungi	When fungi grow in or on living organisms, their hyphae secrete enzymes. These digest substances in the tissues; the products of digestion are absorbed. Growth of hyphae physically damages the tissue. Some fungi also secrete toxins. Others can cause allergic reactions.	Athlete's foot; farmer's lung

Knowledge check 1

Name **two** ways in which pathogens can cause disease.

Effects of lifestyle on the risk of coronary heart disease and cancer

Coronary heart disease usually results from narrowing of the arteries due to atherosclerosis (pp. 52–53). The main risk factors associated with this are shown in Figure 2.

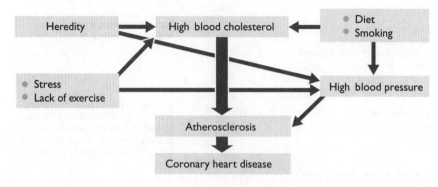

Figure 2 The main risk factors of coronary heart disease (CHD)

Although genetic influences cannot be modified, altering your lifestyle may reduce the extent to which other factors raise the overall risk. The following factors are important:

- taking regular exercise lowers blood pressure, reduces plasma cholesterol levels and reduces resting heart rate
- eating less saturated fat (usually animal fat) reduces the rate at which atherosclerosis develops
- stopping smoking reduces blood pressure
- drinking alcohol only in moderation reduces blood pressure and atherosclerosis

Because several factors influence the risk of coronary heart disease, the cause of the condition is said to be **multifactorial**.

Cancers result from the uncontrolled division of cells — these are covered in Unit 2. Cancers can be fatal if tumour cells spread to other parts of the body, giving rise to 'secondary' cancers that affect the functioning of key organs.

Different cancers have different causes. A higher incidence of breast cancer is linked to several factors including hormone replacement therapy and having children later in life. The incidence of lung cancer is correlated with smoking. The two curves in Figure 3 are similar, but with a time lag of 20 years — the time it takes for lung cancer to develop.

Knowledge check 2

Name **three** changes in lifestyle by which someone could reduce their blood pressure.

examiner tip

When asked in unit tests to describe a graph, you should describe the overall trend or pattern. An appropriate description of the curve for lung cancer in Figure 3 is: 'The deaths from lung cancer increased from 5 deaths per 100 000 in 1920 to 180 deaths per 100 000 in 1975. The increase was slow at first, rapid from 1935 and then slowed after 1975'.

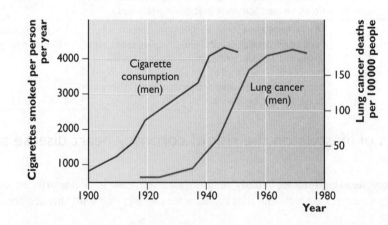

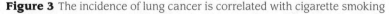

Figure 3 The incidence of lung cancer is correlated with cigarette smoking

Using knowledge and scientific investigations

The correlation between smoking and lung cancer led scientists to believe that something in cigarette smoke caused lung cancer. They could not claim cause and effect because there were uncontrolled variables in the data. However, the correlation led scientists to design investigations to determine the precise cause. Experiments eventually showed that some of the chemicals in cigarette smoke cause mutations in tumour suppressor genes. These genes, in their natural (unmutated) state, normally stop (suppress) the development of a tumour. When the genes mutate, tumours continue to develop and cancers form. The link between cause and effect was established.

The process of establishing a causative agent varies, but Figure 4 gives some idea of the steps that may be involved.

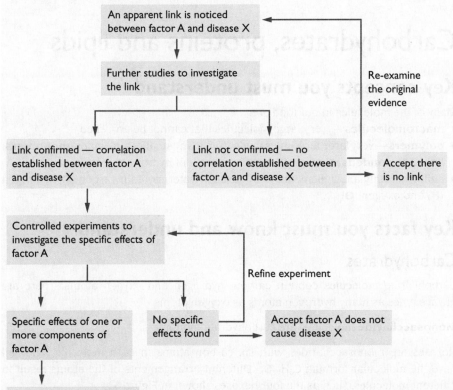

Figure 4 Investigating whether a correlation results from a causal relationship

examiner tip
You might be asked to interpret data that relate a risk factor to the incidence of a specific disease. Be careful not to go beyond what the data show. Only experiments that control confounding variables can establish a causative agent.

Summary

After studying this topic, you should be able to:

- describe how disease can be caused by pathogens penetrating any of an organism's interfaces with the environment
- state that pathogens include bacteria, viruses and fungi
- explain that pathogens cause disease by damaging cells of the host or by releasing toxins
- explain that disease can be caused by the effects of lifestyle
- analyse and interpret data associated with specific risk factors and the incidence of disease
- explain the difference between a correlation and a causal relationship

The molecules in our food

Carbohydrates, proteins and lipids

Key concepts you must understand

Many of the molecules in our food are:

- **macromolecules** — very large molecules that cannot be absorbed
- **polymers** — very large molecules made from many smaller molecules (**monomers**) linked by **condensation** reactions (the reverse of hydrolysis)
- built from only a few elements — all (except water) contain carbon (**C**), hydrogen (**H**) and oxygen (**O**)

Key facts you must know and understand

Carbohydrates

Carbohydrate molecules contain carbon, hydrogen and oxygen atoms. There are always twice as many hydrogen atoms as oxygen atoms.

Monosaccharide molecules are carbohydrate monomers.

Hexoses are monosaccharides with six carbon atoms in each molecule. They all have the molecular formula $C_6H_{12}O_6$. Different arrangements of the atoms result in different molecules, such as the four hexoses shown in Figure 5.

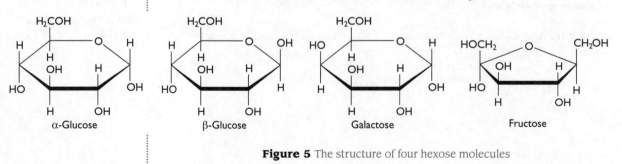

Figure 5 The structure of four hexose molecules

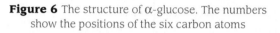

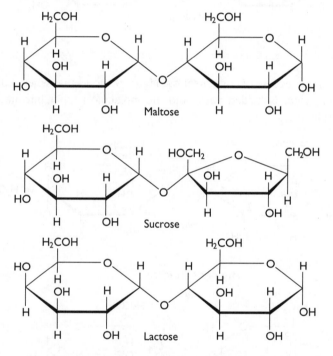

Figure 6 The structure of α-glucose. The numbers
show the positions of the six carbon atoms

examiner tip
You are not expected to
be able to recall these
diagrams. You might,
however, be asked to
draw a simplified diagram
of α-glucose, like the one
shown in Figure 6.

Disaccharide molecules are formed from two monosaccharide molecules linked together by a **glycosidic bond**. Three disaccharides — maltose, sucrose and lactose — are shown in Figure 7.

Figure 7 The structure of three disaccharides

Knowledge check 3
Use Figures 5 and 7 to
name the monosaccharides
joined together in a
molecule of (a) maltose,
(b) sucrose and (c) lactose.

When two monosaccharides combine to form a disaccharide, a molecule of water (H_2O) is formed from a hydroxyl group from one monosaccharide and a hydrogen atom from the other. This allows a bond to be formed that holds the monosaccharides together. The process is called **condensation** and is illustrated in Figure 8.

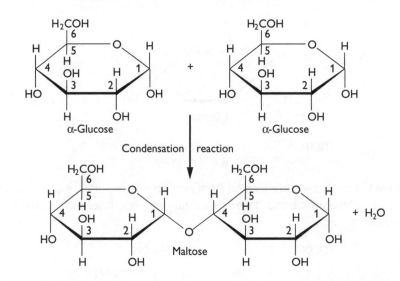

Figure 8 A condensation reaction forms maltose from two molecules of α-glucose

Hydrolysis is the reverse of condensation. Figure 9 shows that when a disaccharide is hydrolysed, water is 'added back' and the molecule is split into its component α-glucose molecules.

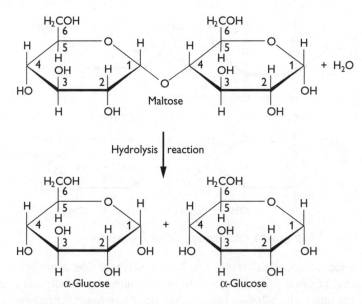

Figure 9 Hydrolysis of maltose forms two molecules of α-glucose

The bond that is broken in Figure 9 is called an **α-1,4-glycosidic bond** because:
- it joins two molecules of α-glucose
- it joins carbon atom **1** of one glucose molecule and carbon atom **4** of the other

The biological basis of related disease

Lactose intolerance

Lactose intolerance arises because many people cannot digest lactose (the disaccharide found in milk and other dairy products) into glucose and galactose.

The enzyme lactase, which hydrolyses lactose, is present in all young humans. By the age of about 4 years, by which time breast-feeding has usually ended, the gene encoding lactase is normally switched off.

In the absence of lactase, undigested lactose passes into the large intestine, where it is fermented by bacteria. This produces small, soluble molecules and gases, such as carbon dioxide and methane. The small, soluble molecules lower the water potential in the large intestine. As a result, water moves into the large intestine by osmosis, causing diarrhoea. The gases cause bloating, cramps and flatulence.

Although more people in the world are lactose-intolerant than are lactose-tolerant, most Europeans remain lactose-tolerant.

examiner tip
Do not confuse lactose and lactase in an examination. The ending 'ose' tells you the molecule is a carbohydrate; the ending 'ase' tells you the molecule is an enzyme.

Polysaccharide molecules are formed from many monosaccharides joined by glycosidic bonds. **Starch** is a common polysaccharide in our diet. You will learn more about its structure, and how its structure is related to its function, in Unit 2.

Proteins

Protein molecules contain the elements carbon, hydrogen and oxygen (as do carbohydrates). They also all contain nitrogen and most contain sulfur.

Proteins have a range of functions. For example, they are important in:
- the structure of **plasma membranes** — protein molecules form ion channels, carrier proteins and surface receptors, e.g. for hormones
- the **immune system** — antibody molecules are proteins
- the **enzymic control** of metabolism — most enzymes are proteins
- the structure of **chromosomes** — DNA is wound around molecules of the protein histone to form a chromosome in eukaryotic cells

Protein molecules are macromolecules because they are polymers of amino acids. **Amino acid** molecules have a carbon atom to which is attached:
- a hydrogen atom
- an amino group (NH_2)
- a carboxyl group (COOH)
- an 'R' group, shown in Figure 10; this represents the other atoms in the molecule and could be a single hydrogen atom, a hydrocarbon chain or a more complex structure

Two amino acids can be joined together by condensation to form a **dipeptide**. The bond that holds the two amino acids together is a **peptide bond**. A **polypeptide** can be formed by the addition of more amino acid molecules. The formation and hydrolysis of a dipeptide is shown in Figure 11.

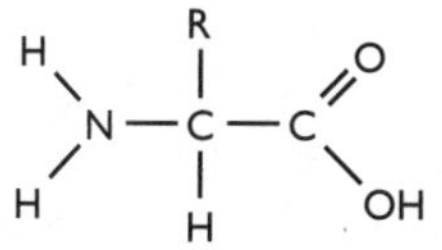

Figure 10 The general structure of an amino acid

Knowledge check 5

Name the type of bond holding together the monomers in
(a) a disaccharide and
(b) a protein.

You might be asked in a unit test to show how two monomers join together by a condensation reaction. Don't forget to show in your answer the water molecule that is formed. Many students fail to gain a mark as a result of this simple omission.

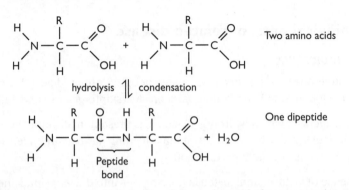

Figure 11 A condensation reaction forms a dipeptide from two amino acids

Figure 12 shows the different 'levels of organisation' in a protein molecule. The sequence of amino acids in the polypeptide is the **primary structure** of the protein. This folds itself into a **secondary structure**, which is either an α-**helix** or a β-**pleated sheet**. Further folding of the molecule produces the **tertiary structure** of the molecule. The tertiary structure of each protein gives the protein molecule a unique shape (either globular or fibrous) and a specific function. For example, it is the specific shape that ensures that:

- the active site of an enzyme molecule can only bind with one substrate
- an insulin receptor in a plasma membrane only binds with insulin
- an antibody molecule only binds with one antigen

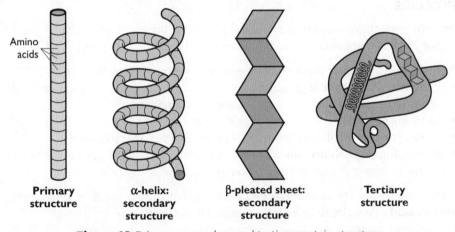

Figure 12 Primary, secondary and tertiary protein structure

Level	Bonds holding structure in place	Description	Notes
Primary	Peptide bonds	Sequence of amino acids in the polypeptide chain	Determined by sequence of triplets of bases in DNA
Secondary	Hydrogen bonds	α-helix or β-pleated sheet	Formed by folding polypeptide chain; both types can exist in the same protein molecule
Tertiary	Ionic, hydrogen and disulfide bridges	Globular or fibrous structure	Gives molecule a unique shape and specific function

Some proteins have one further level of organisation — a **quaternary** structure. Two or more polypeptides are bonded together to form the final protein. Figure 13 shows that a haemoglobin molecule consists of four globular polypeptides (two α-chains and two β-chains) and a collagen molecule contains three fibrous polypeptides.

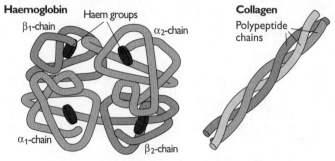

Figure 13 Haemoglobin and collagen are proteins with a quaternary structure

Lipids

Lipid molecules contain atoms of carbon, hydrogen and oxygen, but much less oxygen than in molecules of carbohydrates. The two main types of lipid are:

- **triglyceride** — a glycerol molecule is joined to three fatty acid molecules by ester bonds; triglycerides are used as an energy source in cells
- **phospholipid** — a glycerol molecule is joined to two fatty acids and one phosphate group; phospholipids are used to make plasma membranes

Figure 14 shows the formation and hydrolysis of a triglyceride and the structure of a phospholipid.

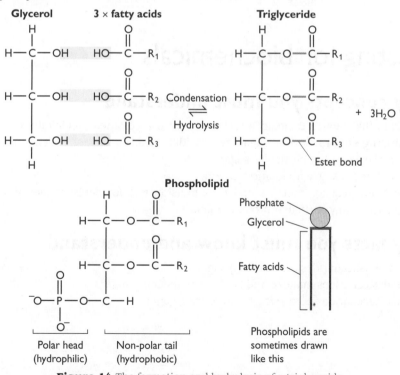

Figure 14 The formation and hydrolysis of a triglyceride and the structure of a phospholipid

Knowledge check 6

Haemoglobin has a quaternary structure. Use Figure 13 to explain why.

Knowledge check 7

Is a lipid molecule a polymer? Explain your answer.

The fatty acids found in triglycerides can be either:

- **saturated fatty acids** — all the carbon–carbon bonds in the molecule are single bonds
- **unsaturated fatty acids** — one or more of the carbon–carbon bonds is a double bond

The difference between saturated and two types of unsaturated fatty acid is shown in Figure 15.

examiner tip

Examiners find that many candidates cannot clearly describe the difference between a saturated and unsaturated fatty acid. You should write that all the carbon atoms are linked by single bonds in a saturated fatty acid or that double bonds occur between some carbon atoms in an unsaturated fatty acid.

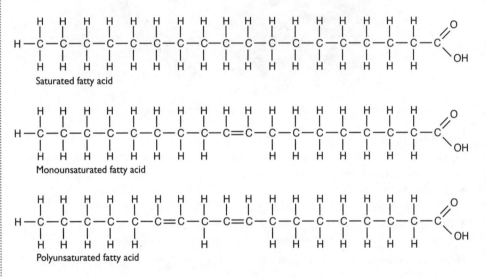

Figure 15 Saturated and unsaturated fatty acids

Testing for biochemicals

Key concepts you must understand

- Sugars that reduce Benedict's reagent to form a coloured precipitate are called **reducing sugars**. Several sugars react with Benedict's reagent, so it cannot show the presence of any particular sugar.
- Only starch reacts with iodine solution.
- The biuret test for proteins and the emulsion test for lipids cannot show the presence of any particular protein or lipid.

Key facts you must know and understand

- All monosaccharides are reducing sugars.
- The disaccharides maltose and lactose are reducing sugars.
- The disaccharide sucrose is a non-reducing sugar.

The biochemical tests you must know are shown in the following table.

Food substance	Reagent	How test is carried out	Result/conclusion
Starch	Iodine solution	Add iodine solution to substance in a test tube or on a white tile	Blue-black colour — starch present; brown colour — starch absent
Reducing sugar	Benedict's solution	Heat substance with Benedict's solution in a test tube in a water bath at 85°C for 5 minutes	Orange/red colour — reducing sugar present; blue/green colour — reducing sugar absent
Non-reducing sugar	Benedict's solution, hydrochloric acid, sodium hydrogen-carbonate	Carry out Benedict's test on food substance in solution; if negative, hydrolyse food solution by boiling with acid; add sodium hydrogencarbonate to neutralise; re-test with Benedict's solution	Initial green colour followed by orange/red colour on re-test — non-reducing sugar present; green on re-test — non-reducing sugar absent
Lipid	Ethanol and water	Add ethanol to food substance in a test tube and shake; filter off any solids; pour the alcohol into a second test tube containing water	White/milky emulsion — lipid present; water remains colourless — lipid absent
Protein	Biuret reagent	Add biuret reagent to food substance in test tube; allow to stand for 5 minutes	Mauve/purple colour — protein present; blue colour — protein absent

> **examiner tip**
> The most common mistake candidates make when describing the test for reducing sugars is to forget that the mixture must be heated. If you don't write that the mixture is heated, you will fail to gain one of the marks available.

After studying this topic, you should be able to:

- recognise the structural formula of the following molecules: α-glucose, a general amino acid, a triglyceride and a phospholipid
- use diagrams to show condensation and hydrolysis reactions involving disaccharides, dipeptides and triglycerides
- distinguish between the primary, secondary, tertiary and quaternary structures of proteins
- describe the protocol for, and positive results of, tests for reducing sugars, non-reducing sugars, starch, lipids and proteins
- explain the biological basis of lactose intolerance

Summary

The structure and functioning of the digestive system

The process of digestion

Key concepts you must understand

- The gut wall is a barrier to absorption of food materials. Most of the molecules **ingested** (taken in) are too large to pass through the gut wall and enter the bloodstream without first being **digested**.
- Digestion involves **hydrolysis reactions** in which large molecules are broken down into smaller ones by adding water molecules (*hydro* = water, *lysis* = splitting).
- The enzymes that catalyse these reactions are **hydrolytic enzymes**. The principle of hydrolysis is illustrated in Figure 16.

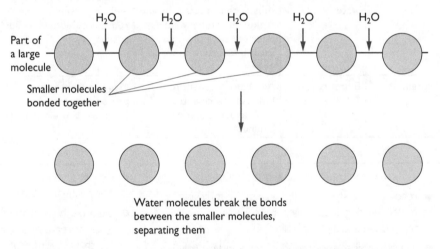

Figure 16 Digestion involves the hydrolysis of polymers into monomers

- The smaller molecules are then **absorbed** and either **respired** (release energy for body functions) or **assimilated** (become part of the body). Molecules that cannot be absorbed are **egested** in the **faeces**.

Key facts you must know and understand

The gut (digestive system) is essentially a tube within the body that opens to the environment at both ends — the mouth and the anus. Several glands are connected to the gut by ducts. Various secretions pass from the glands into the gut along these ducts. Figure 17 is a simplified diagram of the human digestive system.

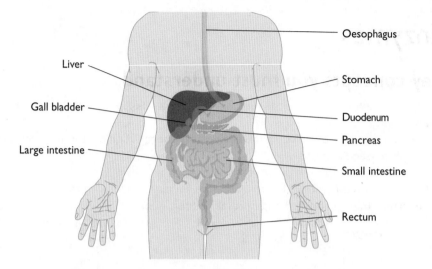

Figure 17 Gross structure of the human digestive system

How starch is digested

Starch is a macromolecule. It cannot cross the gut wall into the bloodstream. It is first digested into the α-glucose monomers from which it is made. This hydrolysis takes place in two stages:

- starch → maltose
- maltose → α-glucose

The hydrolysis of starch into maltose is catalysed by the enzyme **amylase**; the hydrolysis of maltose into α-glucose is catalysed by the enzyme **maltase**.

Amylase is produced by:

- the salivary glands, which secrete (salivary) amylase into the buccal cavity (mouth)
- the pancreas, which secretes (pancreatic) amylase into the duodenum (the upper part of the small intestine)

Maltase is produced by the epithelial cells that line the ileum (the lower part of the small intestine). The enzyme molecules are located in the plasma membranes of these cells. The table below summarises the digestion of starch.

Stage in digestion	Enzyme involved	Notes on reaction
Starch to maltose	Amylase from salivary glands and pancreas	• Amylase catalyses the hydrolysis of α-1,4-glycosidic bonds between α-glucose units in the starch molecule • Optimum pH is neutral to slightly alkaline • Reaction begins in the buccal cavity and recommences in the duodenum • Acid pH of the stomach denatures salivary amylase
Maltose to glucose	Maltase in the plasma membranes of the epithelial cells lining the ileum	• Enzymes in the plasma membrane of cells forming the microvilli hydrolyse α-1,4-glycosidic bonds between the two α-glucose units in maltose molecules • Optimum pH is slightly alkaline

Knowledge check 8

Starch cannot be absorbed unless it is first digested. Explain why.

examiner tip

Be careful to read the precise wording of examination questions. The following questions look similar but require completely different answers.

Q1 Starch is digested to α-glucose in the human gut. Describe how. (6 marks)

Q2 Starch is digested to α-glucose in the human gut. Explain the advantage of this digestion. (3 marks)

Enzymes

Key concepts you must understand

Almost all enzymes are globular proteins that act as biological **catalysts**. Like all catalysts, they:

- speed up reactions by reducing the **activation energy** required for the reaction to take place (see Figure 18)
- are unchanged at the end of the reaction
- do not affect the nature of the reaction (the same products with the same energy are formed in the catalysed and uncatalysed reaction)

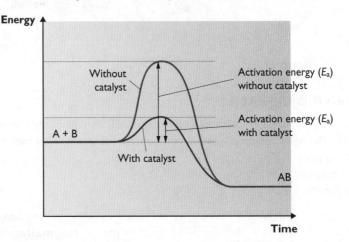

Figure 18 Enzymes reduce the activation energy required for the reaction A + B → AB

Every enzyme has a region called its **active site** that is able to bind with a certain substance (the **substrate**). Because each enzyme has a unique shape, the shape of its active site is unique and can bind with only one substrate; the enzyme is **specific**.

There are two models to explain how enzymes work — the '**lock-and-key**' model and the '**induced-fit**' model. Both models suggest that the active site of the enzyme binds with the substrate to form an **enzyme–substrate complex** (ES complex) and that the formation of this complex reduces the activation energy to allow the reaction to proceed more quickly.

In the lock-and-key model of enzyme action, shown in Figure 19:

- the active site and substrate have **complementary shapes** (like an egg and an egg cup)
- the substrate 'fits' into the active site and binds with it to form an enzyme–substrate complex
- after the reaction, the products leave the active site

Knowledge check 9

Enzymes are protein molecules with a tertiary structure. Why is their tertiary structure important?

Lock-and-key hypothesis

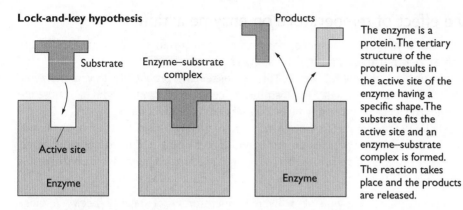

The enzyme is a protein. The tertiary structure of the protein results in the active site of the enzyme having a specific shape. The substrate fits the active site and an enzyme–substrate complex is formed. The reaction takes place and the products are released.

Figure 19 The active site of an enzyme has a fixed shape in the lock-and-key model

In the induced-fit model of enzyme action, shown in Figure 20:

- initially, the shape of the active site is *not quite* complementary to that of the substrate
- as the active site begins to bind, it changes shape and 'moulds' itself around the substrate molecule (like a sock on a foot)
- after the reaction, the products leave the active site and the active site reverts to its original shape

Induced-fit hypothesis

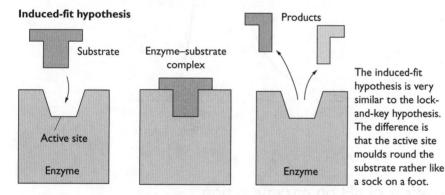

The induced-fit hypothesis is very similar to the lock-and-key hypothesis. The difference is that the active site moulds round the substrate rather like a sock on a foot.

Figure 20 The active site of an enzyme changes to accommodate the substrate in the induced-fit model

The induced-fit model is the preferred model because it better explains the effect of non-competitive inhibitors (described on p. 26).

Key facts you must know and understand

Digestive enzymes constitute only a tiny fraction of the enzymes that exist. Nearly all the reactions that take place in living cells are catalysed by enzymes. The activity of enzymes is affected by:

- temperature
- pH
- substrate concentration
- competitive inhibitors
- non-competitive inhibitors

examiner tip

Candidates make many mistakes when describing enzyme action. They wrongly tell examiners that:

- the active site is on the substrate ✗
- the active site and the substrate have the same shape ✗

Make sure you don't make these mistakes yourself.

Knowledge check 10

An enzyme molecule is specific to one substrate. Use the lock-and-key model of enzyme action to explain why.

The effect of temperature on enzyme action

When the temperature is raised, enzyme molecules and substrate molecules are given more **kinetic energy**, which has two main effects.

- Molecules move around faster. This increases the probability that an enzyme molecule will collide with a substrate molecule and form an enzyme–substrate complex. Overall, more enzyme–substrate complexes will form.
- Particles *within* a molecule vibrate more energetically. This puts strain on the bonds that hold the atoms in place. Bonds begin to break and, in the case of an enzyme, the shape of the active site begins to change. The enzyme begins to **denature**. It is now more difficult for the substrate to bind with the active site.

The activity of an enzyme at a given temperature is a balance between these two effects. The temperature at which an enzyme is most active is its **optimum temperature** (37°C for most human enzymes). Figure 21 summarises the effect of temperature on enzyme activity.

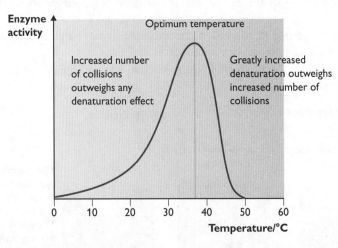

Figure 21 The effect of temperature on enzyme activity

Knowledge check 11

Name the **two** opposing effects of temperature that cause an enzyme to have an optimum temperature.

The effect of pH on enzyme action

The pH scale ranges from 0 to 14. Solutions with a pH of less than 7 are acidic; solutions with a pH of more than 7 are alkaline; a solution with a pH of exactly 7 is neutral.

Most enzymes in humans have an optimum pH within the pH range 6.0–8.0, although the optimum pH of pepsin (an enzyme found in the stomach) is between pH 1.0 and pH 3.0.

Significant changes in pH can affect an enzyme molecule by:

- breaking ionic bonds that hold the protein's tertiary structure in place, leading to denaturation of the enzyme molecule
- altering the charge on some of the amino acids that form the active site, making it more difficult for substrate molecules to bind

These effects occur if the pH becomes either more acidic or more alkaline. Figure 22 shows the effect of pH on enzyme activity.

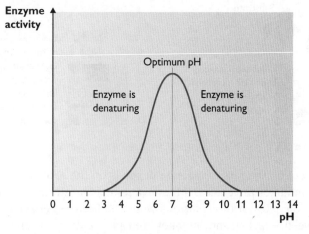

Figure 22 The effect of pH on enzyme activity

The effect of substrate concentration on enzyme activity

A small number of substrate molecules means that there will be relatively few collisions with enzyme molecules and few enzyme–substrate complexes formed. Therefore, the rate of reaction will be slow. Increasing the concentration of the substrate means more collisions and more enzyme–substrate complexes. Eventually, a situation could be reached in which each active site is binding continually with substrate molecules and there is no 'spare capacity' in the system. Increasing the substrate concentration beyond this point cannot increase the activity of the enzyme or the rate of reaction because, at any one moment, all the active sites are occupied. This explains the shape of the curve shown in Figure 23.

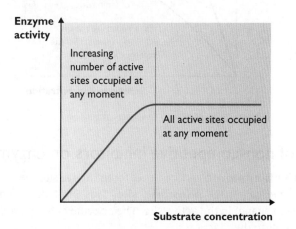

Figure 23 The effect of substrate concentration on enzyme activity

examiner tip
Graphs with a curve of the shape shown in Figure 23 are common in biology. In unit tests, candidates often think they recognise the graph because of this shape and give an answer they have learnt when revising a past question. You must read the labels on the axes of graphs before attempting to answer the questions.

The effect of competitive inhibitors on enzyme activity

Competitive inhibitors have molecules with shapes that are complementary to all, or part, of the active site of an enzyme. They are often similar in shape to the substrate molecules. Figure 24 shows a competitive inhibitor binding temporarily with the active site and preventing substrate molecules from binding.

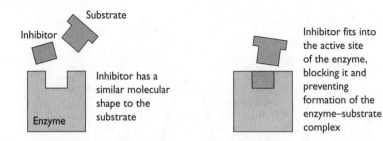

Figure 24 A competitive inhibitor blocks the active site of an enzyme

The overall effect on the rate of reaction depends on the relative concentrations of substrate and inhibitor molecules. If there were nine substrate molecules for every inhibitor molecule, 90% of the collisions would be between enzyme and substrate and 10% between enzyme and inhibitor. Ten per cent of the enzyme molecules would be inhibited and the reaction would proceed at 90% of the maximum rate (at this concentration of the substrate). If there were four substrate molecules to each inhibitor molecule, there would be 20% inhibition and the reaction rate would be 80% of maximum. Figure 25 shows the effect of substrate concentration on inhibition by a fixed concentration of competitive inhibitor.

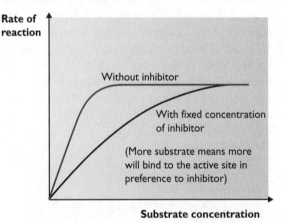

Figure 25 A competitive inhibitor is less effective at higher concentrations of substrate

The effect of non-competitive inhibitors on enzyme action

Non-competitive inhibitors do not compete for the active site — they bind to another part of the enzyme called the **allosteric site**. This produces a **conformational change** (change in shape) in the active site. The enzyme can no longer bind with the substrate and catalyse the reaction.

The effect of a non-competitive inhibitor is not affected by the concentration of the substrate because a non-competitive inhibitor does not bind to the same part of the enzyme. If there are enough inhibitor molecules to bind with the allosteric sites of 80% of the enzyme molecules, then 80% of the enzyme molecules will be inhibited (irrespective of the number of substrate molecules). The reaction rate will drop to

20% of maximum. Figure 26 shows the effect of substrate concentration on inhibition by a fixed concentration of non-competitive inhibitor.

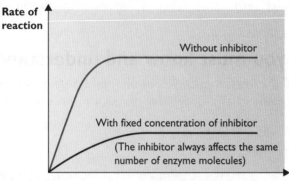

Figure 26 The effect of a non-competitive inhibitor on enzyme activity is not affected by substrate concentration

Summary

After studying this topic, you should be able to:

- explain why macromolecules must be hydrolysed in the gut
- describe how starch is digested in the human gut
- describe the properties of enzymes
- describe the 'lock-and-key' and 'induced-fit' models of enzyme action
- use the models of enzyme action to explain the effect on enzymes of temperature, pH, and concentrations of substrate, competitive inhibitor and non-competitive inhibitor
- interpret graphs showing the effect of the above factors on the rate of enzyme-controlled reactions

Cell structure and the absorption of the products of digestion

Microscopes

Key concepts you must understand

Microscopes produce magnified images of objects.

The detail that can be seen through a microscope does not just depend on the magnification; it also depends on the resolution of the image. **Resolution** is the ability to produce separate images of two points that are close together in an object. If the microscope cannot resolve two points, they are seen as one and detail is lost.

examiner tip
An examiner will
not penalise you for
referring to an optical
microscope (the term in
the specification) as a light
microscope, if you find it
easier to remember.

Electron microscopes have a greater resolving power than optical microscopes because electrons have a shorter wavelength than light. As a result, electron microscopes reveal much more detail of cellular ultrastructure than do optical microscopes.

Key facts you must know and understand

Figure 27 shows that optical microscopes and transmission electron microscopes (TEMs) pass a beam of light or electrons through a specimen. The beam is then focused by:

- glass lenses in optical microscopes
- electromagnetic lenses in TEMs

The image produced by an optical microscope is viewed directly; the image produced by a TEM is viewed on a screen.

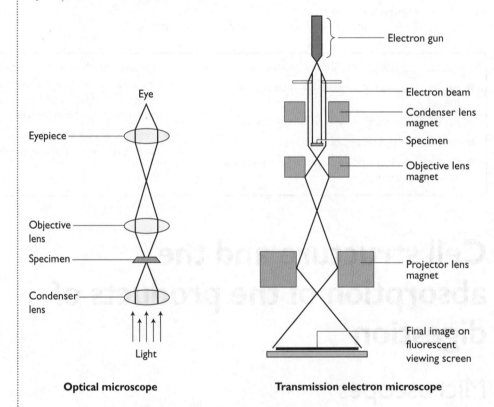

Optical microscope

Transmission electron microscope

Figure 27 The principles of an optical microscope
and a transmission electron microscope

Figure 28 shows that a scanning electron microscope (SEM) directs a beam of electrons at the surface of a specimen and forms an image on a screen from the reflected electrons.

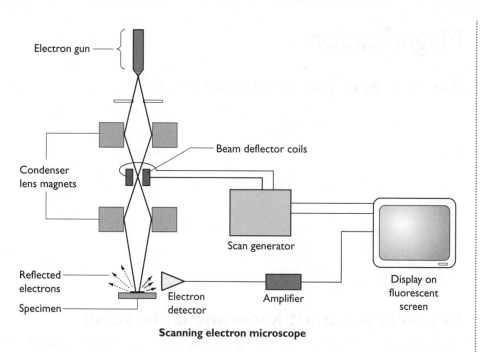

Scanning electron microscope

Figure 28 A scanning electron microscope forms an image from reflected electrons

The main features of the three types of microscope are summarised in the table.

Property	Optical microscope	Transmission electron microscope	Scanning electron microscope
Maximum magnification	1250 times	500 000 times	250 000 times
Focusing	Glass lenses: eyepiece (ocular) lens and objective lens	Electromagnetic lenses	Electromagnetic lenses
Minimum resolution	0.2 μm	1 nm	1 nm
Specimen preparation	Can be mounted in water or aqueous solution; can be alive; may be stained	Specimen is fixed with salts of heavy metals and viewed in a vacuum	Specimen is chemically treated, coated with a thin film of gold and viewed in a vacuum
Image	Viewed directly through the eyepiece	Viewed on a fluorescent screen	Viewed on a fluorescent screen
Limitations	Low resolving power does not allow much subcellular detail to be observed	Specimens are always dead and might contain artefacts as a result of preparation techniques	Specimens are always dead and might contain artefacts as a result of preparation techniques
Advantages	Can be used to view live whole specimens under low magnification	Can produce high-magnification, high-resolution images of cells and organelles	Creates a 3D effect image of the surface of the specimen

Knowledge check 12

Use the table to calculate by how many times the maximum resolving power of the TEM is greater than that of the optical microscope.

Magnification

Key concepts you must understand

Magnification is the ratio between the size of the image (the apparent size) and the size of the object itself (the actual size).

The formula for magnification is:

$$\text{magnification} = \frac{\text{apparent size}}{\text{actual size}}$$

It can be re-written as:

apparent size = actual size × magnification

or

$$\text{actual size} = \frac{\text{apparent size}}{\text{magnification}}$$

Key facts you must know and understand

To use any of these formulae, the apparent size and actual size **must be measured in the same units**. The conversion factors are shown below:

Metres (m)	×1000 ⇌ ÷1000	Millimetres (mm)	×1000 ⇌ ÷1000	Micrometres (μm)	×1000 ⇌ ÷1000	Nanometres (nm)

examiner tip

Candidates often get confused in unit tests when they convert one unit to another unit. You are less likely to make a mistake in a unit test if you make all your measurements in millimetres.

examiner tip

If you have to work out the actual size of an object, always do a common-sense check afterwards. Bacteria are not 3000 mm long!

The structure of epithelial cells from the small intestine

Key concepts you must understand

The structures within a cell are called **organelles**. They can be separated by **cell fractionation**, during which cells are broken up and spun in an ultracentrifuge at varying speeds. This separates the different organelles by mass. The heavier organelles, such as the nuclei, are spun down at low speeds; the lighter ribosomes are spun down at much higher speeds.

The sequence in which the organelles are isolated in decreasing order of mass is:

nuclei – chloroplasts (if plant tissue is used) – mitochondria – lysosomes – ribosomes and membranes (plasma membranes, Golgi apparatus and endoplasmic reticulum)

Tissue for ultracentrifugation is homogenised in a blender using an ice-cold (to reduce enzyme damage), isotonic (to prevent osmotic damage) buffer solution (to stabilise pH).

examiner tip

Be clear in your answer that the solution is isotonic to prevent osmotic damage to the organelles and *not* to the cells. These were seriously damaged when they were burst open by homogenising them in the blender!

Key facts you must know and understand

Figure 29 shows the appearance of an epithelial cell from the small intestine using an optical microscope and using a transmission electron microscope.

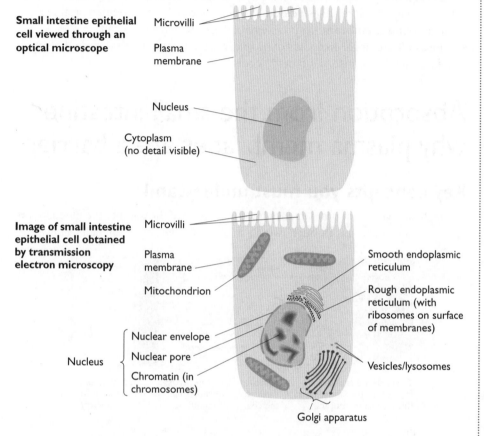

Figure 29 An epithelial cell from the small intestine viewed with an optical microscope and with a TEM

You must learn the functions of the following organelles.

- The **nucleus** contains DNA in the chromatin. The DNA controls protein synthesis through the synthesis of messenger RNA (mRNA); mRNA passes through **pores** in the **nuclear envelope** to reach the cytoplasm.
- **Ribosomes** synthesise proteins by joining amino acids together.
- **Mitochondria** are where aerobic respiration produces ATP, which can release energy for other cellular processes.
- **Lysosomes** contain a mixture of hydrolytic enzymes — they are used to digest old or worn out organelles in the cell or to digest bacteria once engulfed by white blood cells.
- **Rough endoplasmic reticulum (rough ER)** is an internal membrane system with ribosomes attached to it. Proteins made by the ribosomes accumulate in the rough ER and are passed to the Golgi apparatus.

- **Smooth endoplasmic reticulum (smooth ER)** is an internal membrane system without ribosomes attached. It produces steroids and phospholipids, and detoxifies drugs.
- The **Golgi apparatus** modifies proteins (for example by adding carbohydrates to them to make glycoproteins) that are synthesised by the ribosomes and transported by the rough ER. It releases **vesicles** (sacs) containing the modified proteins.
- The **plasma membrane** controls what enters and leaves the cell.
- **Microvilli** are finger-like folds of the plasma membrane that increase the surface area available for absorption of molecules.

Knowledge check 13

How are the functions of the nucleus, rough endoplasmic reticulum and Golgi apparatus linked?

Absorption from the small intestine: why plasma membranes are a barrier

Key concepts you must understand

Figure 30 shows that in order to pass from the lumen of the gut into the bloodstream, digested molecules pass through two plasma membranes of an epithelial cell.

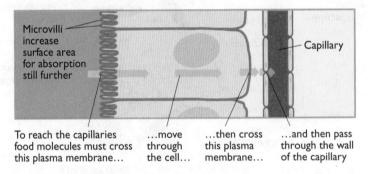

Microvilli increase surface area for absorption still further

Capillary

To reach the capillaries food molecules must cross this plasma membrane...

...move through the cell...

...then cross this plasma membrane...

...and then pass through the wall of the capillary

Figure 30 Absorbed food molecules pass through plasma membranes

Each plasma membrane has the same structure. Scientists believe it is made of a **phospholipid bilayer** with embedded protein molecules. This is known as the **fluid-mosaic** model of membrane structure.

Because the membrane is made largely from phospholipid:
- only small, non-charged molecules (such as oxygen) or lipid-soluble molecules (such as fatty acids) can pass directly through the membrane
- other particles, such as ions (charged particles, such as sodium ions, Na^+, potassium ions, K^+, and calcium ions, Ca^{2+}) and larger non-lipid-soluble molecules (such as glucose and amino acids) must pass through special proteins called **ion channels** (for ions) and **transport proteins** (for other molecules).

This is why the plasma membrane is said to be **partially permeable**.

Key facts you must know and understand

Figure 31(a) gives a 3D impression of the membrane. Figure 31(b) is the kind of representation that you are likely to see in an exam paper.

Knowledge check 14

Explain why the membrane shown in Figure 31 is described as (a) a mosaic and (b) fluid.

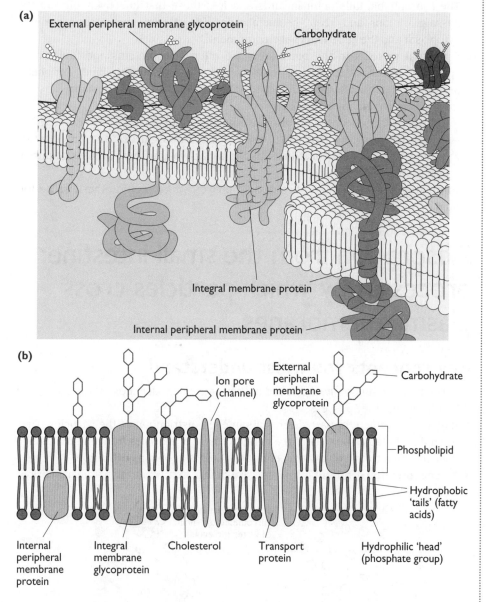

(a)

External peripheral membrane glycoprotein

Carbohydrate

Integral membrane protein

Internal peripheral membrane protein

(b)

Ion pore (channel)

External peripheral membrane glycoprotein

Carbohydrate

Phospholipid

Hydrophobic 'tails' (fatty acids)

Internal peripheral membrane protein

Integral membrane glycoprotein

Cholesterol

Transport protein

Hydrophilic 'head' (phosphate group)

Figure 31 (a) Fluid-mosaic model of the structure of a plasma membrane; (b) simplified version of Figure 31(a)

Notice the two main types of protein in the membrane:

- **peripheral proteins** — sit in just one of the two phospholipid layers
- **integral (transmembrane) proteins** — span both phospholipid layers

The various molecules in the plasma membrane have a number of different functions.

- Phospholipids form a bilayer that gives the membrane its basic structure.
- The hydrophilic (water-loving) heads of the phospholipids point outwards towards the water-containing cytoplasm.
- The hydrophobic tails point inwards and it is these that effectively prevent the passage of ions and keep the membrane distinct from the water-containing cytoplasm and the cell's external environment.
- Peripheral proteins in the outer layer are often glycoproteins and function as specific receptor molecules (e.g. to allow hormone molecules to bind). Peripheral proteins in the inner layer often help to anchor other proteins in position.
- Integral (transmembrane) proteins form:
  - **ion pores** that allow the diffusion of ions in and out of cells
  - **transport proteins** that carry molecules such as glucose and amino acids through membranes (sometimes this is an active transport process requiring energy from ATP)
- **Cholesterol** stabilises the phospholipid bilayer, which would otherwise be too fluid.

Knowledge check 15

Of what are the hydrophobic tails in Figure 31(b) made?

Absorption from the small intestine: processes by which particles cross plasma membranes

Key concepts you must understand

- Particles move randomly; the speed of their movement depends on the amount of kinetic energy they possess.
- Random movement of particles results in even distribution of the particles. They are redistributed as a result of the net movement of particles from an area of high concentration to one of low concentration. This is known as **diffusion**.
- A **concentration gradient** is a progressive change in concentration from high to low.

examiner tip

Think of a concentration gradient as a real gradient — a slope of land from high to low.

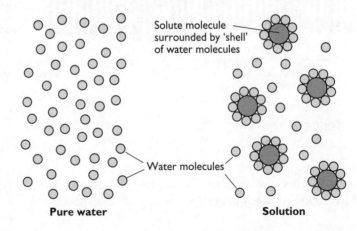

Figure 32 There are more 'free' water molecules in pure water than in a solution

- **Water potential (Ψ)** is a measure of the concentration of free water molecules in a solution. Figure 32 shows that, in pure water, all the molecules are 'free' and so this has the highest water potential; its value is 0 kPa. In solutions, some of the water molecules form a shell around the solute molecules and are no longer free so the water potential is reduced (becomes negative). Concentrated solutions have less free water than dilute solutions and so have lower (more negative) water potentials.
- Diffusion is a process by which particles move freely across a membrane from a high concentration to a low concentration (down the concentration gradient).
- **Facilitated diffusion** is another process by which particles move across a membrane from a high concentration to a low concentration (down the concentration gradient). In facilitated diffusion, the particles either:
  - pass through protein channels (ions)
  or
  - are carried across the membrane by transport proteins (e.g. glucose and amino acids)
- **Active transport** results in particles moving across a membrane from a low concentration to a high concentration (against the concentration gradient). Carrier proteins are always needed, as is hydrolysis of ATP to supply the necessary energy. The carrier proteins are often referred to as **pumps**.
- **Osmosis** is the net movement of water molecules across a partially permeable membrane from a region of high water potential to a region of lower (more negative) water potential.

Key facts you must know and understand

The four main transport processes are compared in the table below.

Process	Movement with respect to concentration gradient	Energy requirement	Types of particles moved across membrane	Transport proteins
Diffusion	Down gradient	Kinetic energy of particles	Lipid soluble; small, non-polar molecules	None
Facilitated diffusion	Down gradient	Kinetic energy of particles	Ions and medium-sized molecules (e.g. glucose)	Protein channels (ions) or carrier proteins (glucose)
Active transport	Against gradient	Hydrolysis of ATP	Ions and medium-sized molecules	Carrier proteins (pumps)
Osmosis	Down water potential gradient	Kinetic energy of particles	Water molecules	None (though some cells have aquaporins that increase water movement)

> **examiner tip**
> Think of rolling a boulder up and down a real gradient. It needs no extra energy to roll down the slope, but if you want to move it back up again (against the gradient), you have to bend your back and use a lot of energy!

> **Knowledge check 16**
> A cell with a water potential of −20 kPa is put into a solution with a water potential of −10 kPa. Will the cell gain or lose water? Explain your answer.

> **examiner tip**
> Never refer to the movement of particles along a concentration gradient. Examiners want you to tell them in which direction the particles move — up or down the concentration gradient.

Absorption from the small intestine: pathways and mechanisms

Key concepts you must understand

- Glucose is absorbed from the small intestine by a mechanism that involves the co-transport (simultaneous transport) of sodium ions.
- The transport protein carries a glucose molecule with a sodium ion into the epithelial cell by facilitated diffusion.
- Facilitated diffusion only works if there is a diffusion gradient. This is maintained by the active transport of sodium ions out of the base of the epithelial cell; glucose molecules pass out by facilitated diffusion.
- Absorption is efficient because:
  - microvilli increase the surface area of the epithelial cells for absorption
  - the distance from the lumen of the intestine to the capillaries is short
  - there is always a concentration gradient between the lumen of the small intestine and the epithelial cells
- For the process of simple diffusion, the relationship between the above points is expressed in the formula:

$$\text{rate of diffusion} \propto \frac{\text{surface area} \times \text{difference in concentration}}{\text{thickness of exchange surface (diffusion distance)}}$$

- For facilitated diffusion, this formula is modified to:

$$\text{rate of diffusion} \propto \frac{\text{number of transport proteins} \times \text{difference in concentration}}{\text{thickness of exchange surface (diffusion distance)}}$$

Key facts you must know and understand

Figure 33 shows the location of some transport proteins and outlines the mechanism of the uptake of sodium ions and of glucose.

Knowledge check 17

In addition to glucose, Figure 33 shows the absorption of amino acids from the small intestine. You are not required to recall the absorption of amino acids. Test your ability to interpret a diagram by using Figure 33 to describe how amino acids are absorbed.

Knowledge check 18

The transport proteins shown in Figure 33 are specific to either glucose or amino acids. Explain how.

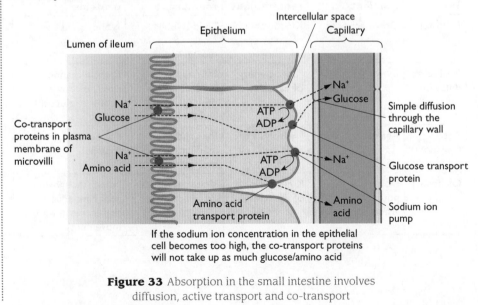

If the sodium ion concentration in the epithelial cell becomes too high, the co-transport proteins will not take up as much glucose/amino acid

Figure 33 Absorption in the small intestine involves diffusion, active transport and co-transport

The biological basis of related disease

Cholera

Cholera is a bacterial disease that affects absorption from the small intestine. Figure 34 shows that, like all bacteria, the bacterium that causes cholera has a prokaryotic cell. Prokaryotic cells differ from the eukaryotic cells of animals, plants and fungi.

- They are usually much smaller.
- They do not have a true nucleus (the DNA is not contained within a nuclear envelope).
- They do not have membrane-bound organelles (i.e. they do not have lysosomes, mitochondria and chloroplasts).
- They have circular DNA (the DNA forms a closed loop rather than being a linear molecule).
- They have 'naked' DNA (the DNA is not associated with proteins in chromosomes).
- They have plasmids (very small circular pieces of DNA).
- The cell wall is made of peptidoglycan (not cellulose like a plant cell wall or chitin like a fungal cell wall).
- Some bacteria have a 'capsule' outside the cell wall.

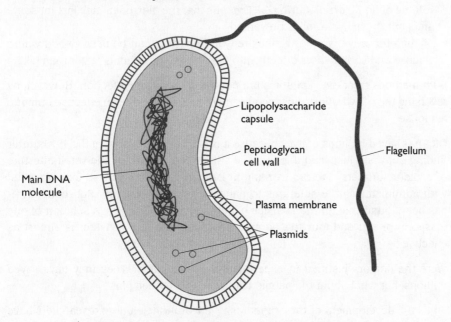

Figure 34 The cholera bacterium (*Vibrio cholerae*)

The cholera bacterium (*Vibrio cholerae*) causes disease in the following way.

- It is transmitted in polluted water.
- In the small intestine, the bacterium anchors itself to the epithelial cells, multiplies and produces a toxin.
- The toxin affects transport proteins in the plasma membrane of the epithelial cells.

- Sodium and chloride ions pass out of the epithelial cells and create a salt-water environment with a low water potential in the lumen of the small intestine. This is ideal for the cholera bacterium, which occurs naturally in salty water.
- Water is lost by osmosis from the cells (and then from the blood) to the lumen of the small intestine, causing:
  - diarrhoea (the production of very watery faeces)
  - massive dehydration
- If not treated in time, the dehydration can be fatal.

Most deaths from cholera occur as a result of dehydration. Oral rehydration therapy (ORT) aims to reverse dehydration and so give the patient time to mount an effective immune response against the bacterium. The aim is to put back into the blood and cells the water and mineral ions lost due to the action of the cholera toxin. It involves giving the patient a solution that contains mainly glucose and sodium ions (as sodium chloride and sodium citrate).

- For ORT, the patient drinks a commercially pre-prepared powder dissolved in water. The glucose and sodium ions in the solution are taken up by co-transport proteins in the plasma membranes of epithelial cells. This increases the concentration of solutes in the cells and in the blood plasma, lowering their water potential. Water follows by osmosis, rehydrating the patient. The sheer volume of liquid drunk during ORT means that the diarrhoea may last for some time, but the dehydration is prevented.
- As an alternative, an intravenous rehydration 'drip' can be used to add water, glucose and sodium ions directly into the plasma. Its effect is faster than ORT.

Both methods treat the symptoms but not the cause of the infection. However, by reversing the dehydration, most people are then able to make an effective immune response.

ORT has saved millions of lives because it is easy to administer. In the 1970s, after finding out that glucose and ions could still be reabsorbed by the small intestine of cholera sufferers, doctors working in Pakistan and Bangladesh experimented with administering the solutions to patients orally (by mouth). Subsequently, it has been found that, in the absence of commercial ORT mixes, a solution of one teaspoon of salt and four teaspoons of sugar in one litre of water is almost as effective.

Were the doctors justified in experimenting on humans? They may have saved millions, but what about the people who were the 'guinea pigs'?

Since the development of the original oral rehydration solution, researchers have found that:

- reducing the glucose and salt concentrations slightly and drinking slightly less is just as effective in rehydrating the patient; it also reduces the diarrhoea more quickly
- including amino acids in the mixture helps in rehydration because amino acids help the absorption of sodium ions through the amino acid–sodium co-transport protein

Knowledge check 19

Why must ORT solutions contain both sodium chloride and glucose?

After studying this topic, you should be able to:

- explain the terms magnification and resolution
- use your understanding of optical and electron microscopes to explain the advantages and limitations of their use
- calculate the actual size of specimens when given information about magnification
- recognise and describe the function of cell organelles
- apply your understanding of cell fractionation and ultracentrifugation to identify organelles
- apply your knowledge of cell organelles to explain how eukaryotic cells are adapted for their functions
- use the fluid-mosaic model to explain the properties of the plasma membrane
- explain the differences between diffusion, facilitated diffusion and active transport
- use your knowledge of osmosis to identify the movement of water between cells and between cells and solutions
- use your understanding of co-transport of glucose with sodium ions to explain the symptoms of cholera and how ORT reduces these symptoms

The lungs, breathing and gas exchange

Key concepts you must understand

The mechanism of breathing

Air moves into and out of the lungs because of pressure differences. Air moves from a region of high pressure to a region of low pressure.

Breathing movements create pressure differences.
- Inhaling creates a lower pressure in the lungs than in the atmosphere and so air moves in.
- Exhaling creates a higher pressure in the lungs than in the atmosphere and so air moves out.

The amount of air we inhale in one minute is the **pulmonary ventilation rate**. It depends on:
- how much air is inhaled in each breath (the **tidal volume**)
- the ventilation rate (number of breaths taken per minute, i.e. breathing rate)

pulmonary ventilation rate = tidal volume × ventilation rate

Gas exchange in the alveoli

Concentration gradients allow oxygen to diffuse from the air in the alveoli into the red blood cells and carbon dioxide to diffuse from the blood plasma into the alveoli.

The high rate of diffusion of gases between the blood and the alveoli can be explained using the formula:

$$\text{rate of diffusion} \propto \frac{\text{surface area} \times \text{difference in concentration}}{\text{thickness of exchange surface (diffusion distance)}}$$

> **examiner tip**
> Think of gas coming out of a gas tap; it does so because the pressure in the gas pipe is greater than air pressure.

> **Knowledge check 20**
> If you know the pulmonary ventilation rate and the breathing rate, how would you find the tidal volume?

- There is a large surface area created by the millions of alveoli.
- There is a steep concentration gradient created by:
  - the circulation bringing blood low in oxygen and high in carbon dioxide to the capillaries around the alveoli
  - ventilation bringing air high in oxygen and low in carbon dioxide into the alveoli
- The alveolar epithelium (the wall of the alveoli) is extremely thin; it is made from squamous epithelium.

The **partial pressure** of a gas in a mixture is the proportion of the total pressure exerted by that gas. It is a way of expressing the concentration of a gas. For example, oxygen makes up 21% of the air, so it exerts 21% of the total atmospheric pressure. The partial pressure of a gas is written, for example, as pO_2, pCO_2 etc.

Knowledge check 21

Explain the advantage of ventilating the lungs.

Key facts you must know and understand

The structure of the human breathing system

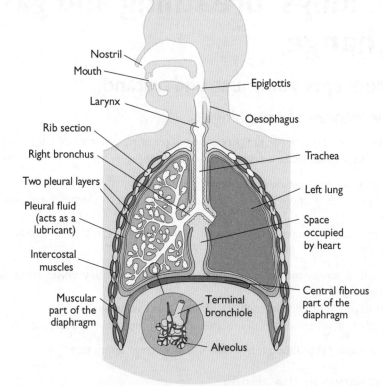

Figure 35 Gross structure of the human gas exchange system

The mechanism of breathing

- Movement of the ribs and diaphragm changes the volume of the thorax.
- **Intercostal muscles** (between the ribs) raise and lower the ribs.
- The external muscular region of the diaphragm raises and lowers the central fibrous region of the diaphragm.

Inhalation

The flowchart in Figure 36 summarises the mechanism of inhalation.

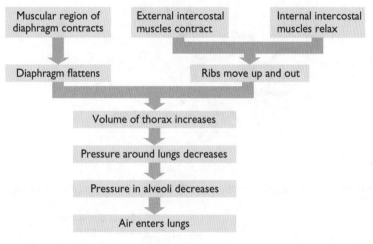

Figure 36 The mechanism of inhalation (breathing in)

Exhalation

The flowchart in Figure 37 summarises the mechanism of exhalation.

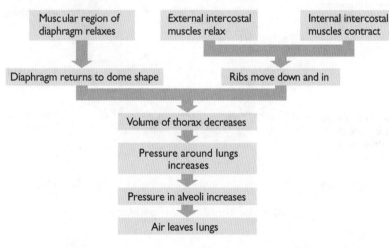

Figure 37 The mechanism of exhalation (breathing out)

Knowledge check 22

Write a description of how muscles cause our breathing movements. It will be good practice for the last question on BIOL1, which always tests AO1. Assume there are 5 marks for this, so you should write five things you have learnt about this subject.

Gas exchange in the alveoli

Figure 38 shows the relationship between bronchioles, alveoli and blood vessels.

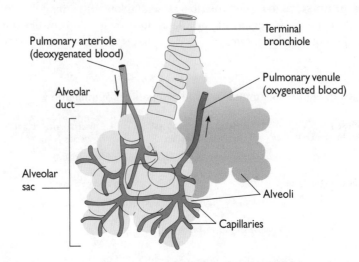

Figure 38 The ends of small bronchioles have alveoli surrounded by blood capillaries

The gas exchange pathways associated with an alveolus are outlined in Figure 39.

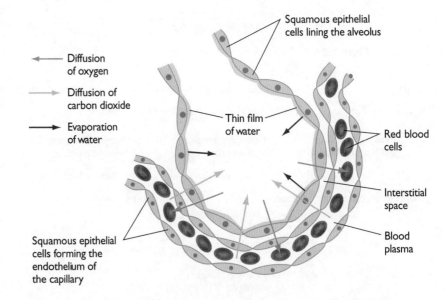

Figure 39 Gas exchange between an alveolus and a blood capillary

The flowcharts in Figure 40 show the diffusion pathways of oxygen and carbon dioxide.

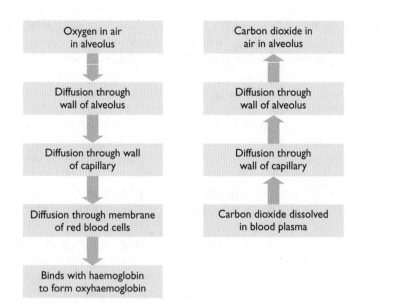

Figure 40 Diffusion pathways of oxygen and carbon dioxide

The biological basis of related disease

Diseases of the lungs

Because the lungs form an interface with the environment, they are affected by:
- microorganisms in the air breathed in
- chemicals in the air breathed in
- solid particles in the air breathed in

Burning plant material slowly and at low temperatures (as in cigarette smoking) produces toxic chemicals, rather than carbon dioxide and water (produced when the same materials are burnt quickly at high temperatures).

Some of the toxic chemicals in cigarette smoke cause mutations (alterations in gene structure and function). Others are oxidants that damage substances in the body that are involved in maintaining a healthy structure of the lungs and blood vessels.

Much of the evidence linking lifestyle conditions with disease stems from a correlation between an environmental factor and an increase in the occurrence of the disease. It does not provide direct evidence of cause and effect.

Pulmonary tuberculosis — a contagious lung disease

Pulmonary tuberculosis is caused by the bacterium *Mycobacterium tuberculosis*.

The bacterium is spread from person to person in droplets produced by sneezing and coughing. When these droplets are inhaled, the disease can progress in different ways, depending on the health of the individual.

- On reaching the alveoli, the bacteria are engulfed by macrophages (similar to phagocytic white blood cells), but not destroyed. They multiply inside the macrophages and eventually cause the macrophages to burst, releasing more bacteria.
- After about 21 days, T cells (see page 55) begin to arrive at the site and activate other macrophages so that they can destroy the bacteria.
- It is at this stage (primary tuberculosis) that the health of the person is critical. Often, the activated macrophages are able to destroy the bacteria and the disease progresses no further. However, if the immune system is weakened, the following can occur.
- The bacteria are not eliminated by the macrophages and the immune system effectively 'walls off' the bacteria in tubercles. These are lumps in the lungs with a semi-solid centre. The bacteria can survive in the tubercle, but do not multiply. They can remain in this condition for many years — people are infected, but show no symptoms and do not infect other people.
- If the bacteria become active again, the tubercles grow and may invade a bronchus (allowing the bacteria to spread to other parts of the lungs) or an artery (allowing the bacteria to spread to other parts of the body and create secondary infections). This is active tuberculosis. The rapid multiplication of the bacteria at this stage results in the formation of cavities in the lung, which gave the disease its common name of 'consumption'.
- Cavities in the lung reduce both the effectiveness of ventilation and the rate of gas exchange in the alveoli.

Symptoms of TB include:
- chest pain and coughing up blood
- a cough that lasts for more than 3 weeks
- chills and fever
- night sweats
- loss of appetite and loss of weight
- fatigue

People most at risk of infection include those who:
- are in regular contact with large numbers of people (e.g. in nursing homes, prisons, schools)
- have an inadequate diet
- inject drugs
- drink alcohol to excess
- are infected by HIV

Emphysema — a chronic obstructive pulmonary disorder

Emphysema is one form of chronic obstructive pulmonary disorder (COPD); it is nearly always the result of cigarette smoking.

Toxins in cigarette smoke provoke an inflammatory response, which leads to the breakdown of the walls of the alveoli. Figure 41 shows how this reduces the area of the gas exchange surface.

Knowledge check 23

How will cavities in the lungs caused by tuberculosis reduce (a) the effectiveness of ventilation and (b) the rate of gas exchange?

Knowledge check 24

Why does an inadequate diet and infection by HIV increase the risk of infection by TB?

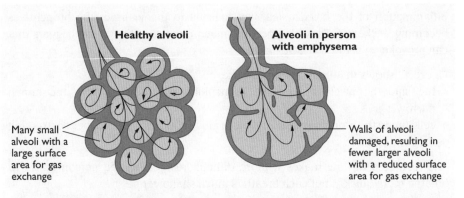

Figure 41 Emphysema reduces the surface area for gas exchange

The amount of elastin (a protein) in the tissues surrounding the airways is also reduced. This makes it more difficult for alveoli that have been stretched by inhaling to recoil to their natural size and force air out. The airflow in and out of the alveoli is reduced.

The overall result is that oxygen uptake by the blood is reduced greatly, so that less is available for the production of ATP in respiration. For a person with advanced emphysema, any activity is a great effort.

Pulmonary fibrosis — a lung disease caused by solid particles

Pulmonary fibrosis is a condition in which the tissue between the bronchioles and alveoli becomes scarred as a result of small solid particles continually entering the lung.

The development of scar tissue in the lungs twists the alveoli and bronchi out of shape, compressing some and stretching others, and reduces the elasticity of the tissue surrounding the airways. As with emphysema, airflow and gas exchange are both reduced, although the cause is different.

Any job which involves producing small solid particles that might be inhaled will increase the risk of fibrosis — for example:
- jobs that involve grinding stone or metal
- working with asbestos — some kinds release small, sharp fibres
- working with mouldy hay — the hyphae of some fungi trigger an inflammatory response that brings about fibrosis; in this case it is known as 'farmer's lung'

Asthma — a lung disease resulting from an allergic response

Asthma is a condition in which the bronchioles become chronically inflamed. Two main factors are thought to be involved:
- a genetic predisposition to asthma
- exposure to certain allergens at an early age (these include tobacco smoke, pollen grains, the faeces of dust mites and other particles that can be inhaled)

In susceptible people, these substances produce an allergic response. White blood cells called mast cells invade the bronchioles and release histamines. This causes

Knowledge check 25

Suggest how the disease miners' lung is caused.

inflammation of the bronchioles, which leads to the walls of the bronchioles becoming thickened. They also become much more sensitive to the triggers that can provoke an asthma attack.

Figure 42 shows that in an asthma attack:
- the smooth muscle around the bronchioles contracts, making the lumen narrower
- cells lining the bronchioles secrete more mucus than normal, further obstructing the flow of air

The restricted airflow makes it more difficult to breathe; the person starts to breathe more quickly, but each breath is much shallower.

As a result of the restricted airflow, gas exchange in the alveoli is reduced.

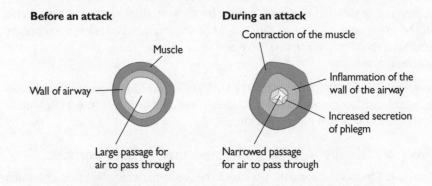

Figure 42 Asthma reduces the lumen of bronchioles

The triggers that can cause an attack in susceptible people include:
- some diseases, particularly the common cold and flu
- exposure to fumes, smoke and dust
- exposure to allergens, such as pollen, animal fur, some medicines and some foods
- exercise — especially in cold, dry air
- emotions (laughing or crying hard) and stress

Summary

After studying this topic, you should be able to:
- recognise the trachea, bronchi, bronchioles, alveoli and related blood vessels in a diagram of the human breathing system
- explain how the structure of the human breathing system is adapted for efficient gas exchange
- show your understanding of how changes in volume and pressure result in ventilation of the lungs
- describe how the activity of the diaphragm muscles and intercostal muscles brings about breathing movements
- use data to calculate pulmonary ventilation
- describe the transmission, symptoms and course of infection of pulmonary tuberculosis
- use your understanding of lung function to explain the effects of asthma, emphysema, fibrosis and tuberculosis on lung function
- interpret data relating specific risk factors and the incidence of lung disease

The structure and functioning of the heart

Key concepts you must understand

- The heart is a muscular pump. Contraction and relaxation of the muscular walls of the chambers of the heart create pressure differences that make the blood flow from regions of high pressure to regions of low pressure.
- **Systole** means that the walls of a chamber are contracting. This raises the pressure of blood in that chamber.
- **Diastole** means that the walls of a chamber are relaxing. This allows the pressure of blood in that chamber to fall.
- Pressure changes open and close valves in the heart, which controls the flow of blood through the heart.
- Humans have a double circulation, as shown in Figure 43. During one complete circulation of the body, the blood passes through the heart twice. It is pumped to the lungs where it is oxygenated (the pulmonary circulation) and then returns to the heart where it is pumped to other parts of the body that use the oxygen (the systemic circulation). This ensures that:
  - blood passing to the tissues is always saturated with oxygen because the pulmonary and systemic circulations are separate
  - blood is delivered to the tissues at high pressure (producing a more efficient circulation) because it is pumped twice by the heart

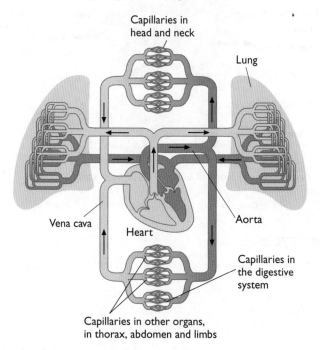

Figure 43 Like all mammals, humans have a double circulation

Knowledge check 26

Distinguish between diastole and systole.

- The heartbeat is **myogenic** — it does not depend on nervous stimulation to beat; it has its own natural pacemaker that triggers each heartbeat.
- The amount of blood pumped from a ventricle when it contracts is the **stroke volume**.
- The number of contractions per minute is the **heart rate**.
- The total amount of blood pumped from a ventricle each minute is the cardiac output = heart rate × stroke volume.

Factors that affect either stroke volume or heart rate affect the cardiac output. These include:
- exercise
- stress
- emotion
- disease

Knowledge check 27

An athlete's cardiac output is 3 dm³ per minute and her heart rate is 60 beats per minute. What is the value of her stroke volume?

Key facts you must know and understand

The structure of the human heart

You should be able to identify the parts of the heart shown in Figures 44 and 45, and able to explain their functions.

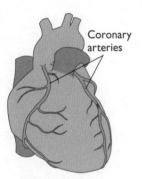

Figure 44 Coronary arteries supply blood to the heart muscle

Knowledge check 28

What will cause the right atrioventricular valve in Figure 45 to close?

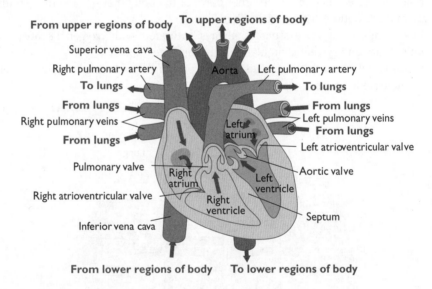

From upper regions of body

To upper regions of body

Superior vena cava

Right pulmonary artery

Aorta

Left pulmonary artery

To lungs

To lungs

From lungs

From lungs

Right pulmonary veins

Left pulmonary veins

Left atrium

From lungs

From lungs

Left atrioventricular valve

Pulmonary valve

Aortic valve

Right atrium

Right atrioventricular valve

Left ventricle

Inferior vena cava

Right ventricle

Septum

From lower regions of body

To lower regions of body

Figure 45 The internal structure of the heart

The cardiac cycle

The main events of the cardiac cycle are shown in Figure 46 and summarised in the table.

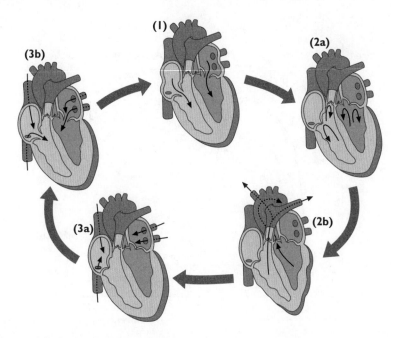

Figure 46 The events of the cardiac cycle are further described in the table below

Stage	Action of atria	Result	Action of ventricles	Result
(1) Atrial systole	Walls contract	Blood forced through valves into ventricles	Walls relax	Ventricles fill with blood
(2) Ventricular systole	Walls relax	Blood neither enters nor leaves atria	Walls contract	(a) Initially no blood leaves, but pressure of blood in ventricles increases (b) Pressure of blood opens valves and blood is ejected into main arteries
(3) Ventricular diastole	Walls relax	(a) Initially, blood enters atria but cannot pass into ventricles as valves still closed (b) As more blood enters atria it forces open valves and passes into ventricles	Walls relax	(a) Blood neither enters nor leaves (b) Blood enters from atria by 'passive ventricular filling' — not due to atrial contraction

Figure 47 shows the pressure changes of blood in the left side of the heart during one cardiac cycle.

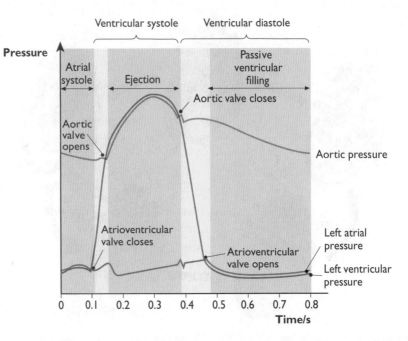

Figure 47 Pressure changes associated with the cardiac cycle

A graph of the changes in the right atrium, right ventricle and pulmonary artery shows all the same features, but all the pressures are lower.

Controlling the cardiac cycle

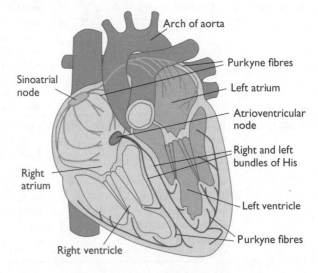

Figure 48 The conducting system of the heart includes the SAN, AVN and Purkyne fibres

AQA AS Biology

- The **sinoatrial node** (**SAN**) is a bundle of cells in the right atrium that generates electrical impulses.
- **Purkyne tissue** consists of fibres of modified cardiac muscle that conduct the impulses generated by the SAN. Purkyne tissue crosses all parts of both atria. In the ventricles, it is organised into two main areas called the **bundles of His**.
- The **atrioventricular node** (**AVN**) is the only place where electrical impulses can pass from atria to ventricles. It conducts impulses only slowly.

Figure 48 shows this electrical conducting system of the heart.

The table summarises the main events involved in controlling the cardiac cycle.

Event in cardiac electrical conducting system	Event in cardiac cycle	Stage of cardiac cycle
The SAN generates an impulse; the impulse spreads along Purkyne fibres to all parts of the atria	Cardiac muscle in atria contracts, cardiac muscle in ventricles is relaxed — blood is forced through AV valves from atria to ventricles	Atrial systole/ ventricular diastole
The impulse is held up at the AVN, allowing time for atria to empty	Cardiac muscle in atria contracts, cardiac muscle in ventricles is relaxed — blood continues to be forced through AV valves	Atrial systole/ ventricular diastole
The impulse is conducted along the bundles of His through the ventricle walls	Cardiac muscle in atria relaxes, cardiac muscle in ventricles contracts; AV valves closed; then aortic/pulmonary valves opened — blood ejected into main arteries	Atrial diastole/ ventricular systole
No impulse	Cardiac muscle in atria and ventricles is relaxed — passive ventricular filling	Atrial and ventricular diastole

Knowledge check 30

Explain the advantage of (a) the delay in the impulses passing through the AVN and (b) the ventricles contracting from their base upwards.

The biological basis of related disease

Coronary heart disease — a multi-factorial condition

Cardiac muscle cells continue to respire efficiently only if they have a constant supply of oxygen and glucose. The energy released is used in the contraction of the chambers of the heart. Oxygen and glucose are carried to the cardiac muscle in the coronary arteries. If the coronary circulation is interrupted (e.g. by a blocked artery):

- part of the wall of the heart is deprived of oxygen and glucose
- the cells in this region cannot respire and release energy
- the muscle in this region will be unable to contract

This may cause the heart to stop beating — a myocardial infarction or heart attack.

Figure 49 shows the effect of a blocked heart artery.

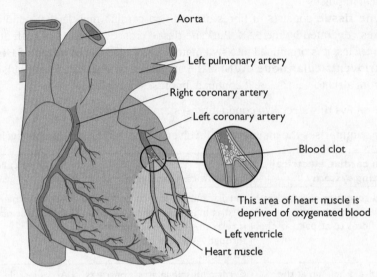

Figure 49 Blockage of a coronary artery leads to death of heart muscle and sometimes to myocardial infarction

Atherosclerosis is a process in which atheroma (a mixture of fatty substances including cholesterol, cells and fibres of connective tissue) is deposited in walls of arteries. Figure 50 shows how atherosclerosis narrows an artery and roughens its inner lining (endothelium). This can have several consequences.

- A blood clot is more likely to form in the artery because a roughened surface triggers clot formation.
- The artery is more likely to become blocked by a blood clot because it is already narrowed by the atheroma.

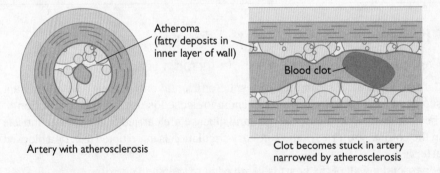

Figure 50 Atheroma in the wall of an artery leads to atherosclerosis

- An aneurysm may develop; the atheroma weakens the wall of the artery and the pressure of the blood distends the artery (Figure 51).
- If the aneurysm bursts then blood will be lost.
  - Blood loss from even a small aneurysm in the brain can put pressure on the brain and cause a stroke.
  - Blood loss from a large aneurysm in the aorta is nearly always fatal.

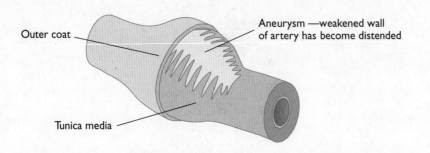

Figure 51 Aneurysm — distension of an artery wall weakened by atheroma

A number of factors influence the rate and extent of atherosclerosis. These are shown in Figure 2 on page 10.

After studying this topic, you should be able to:

- relate the gross structure of the heart and its associated blood vessels to heart function
- show understanding of how pressure changes in the heart chambers result in valve movements and changes in blood flow by interpreting data relating to the cardiac cycle
- calculate cardiac output, heart rate or stroke volume when given the values of any two of these variables
- show understanding of the roles of the SAN, AVN and Purkyne tissue in the myogenic control of the heartbeat
- describe how atheroma develops within the walls of arteries and contributes to an increased risk of thrombosis and aneurysm
- describe the causes and effects of myocardial infarction
- interpret data relating the incidence of coronary heart disease with diet, blood cholesterol, cigarette smoking and high blood pressure

Summary

The body's reaction to infection

Key concepts you must understand

Antigens are usually glycoproteins on the surface of cells. Foreign antigens (those that are not found on our own cells) trigger an **immune response** that is specific to that antigen.

An **antibody** is a protein with a complementary shape to a particular antigen. It can bind with this antigen to form an **antigen–antibody complex**. Figure 52 shows that, although all antibodies have the same basic shape, each has a unique variable region that allows it to be specific to a single antigen.

Knowledge check 31

How is a glycoprotein different from a protein?

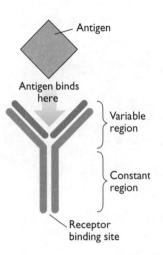

Figure 52 All antibody molecules have two long and two short polypeptide chains

Each pathogen has one or more different antigens on its surface, each of which triggers a different specific immune response when the pathogen infects us.

There are two types of specific immune response.
- There is a response to antigens of bacteria, viruses and toxins that are exposed in the bloodstream. This is the **humoral response**. It involves the release of **antibodies** by **B lymphocytes** (**B cells**). Before they are activated, the B cells display their antibodies on their cell surfaces.
- There is a response to foreign antigens on the surface of our own cells that are infected by viruses or are cancerous. This is the **cell-mediated response**, brought about by **T lymphocytes** (**T cells**).

The humoral response and the cell-mediated response both depend on an initial recognition process by white blood cells called **macrophages**.

The initial immune response to a foreign antigen is called a **primary immune response**. It destroys the microorganisms or toxins and creates **memory cells**. These cells have an **immunological memory** and 'recognise' the same antigen if it enters the body again. They then mount a **secondary immune response**. This is quicker and more effective than the primary response as the memory cells are present in larger numbers than the original inactive lymphocytes.

As a result:
- memory B cells form antibody-secreting plasma cells in greater numbers and more quickly, and release antibodies in much higher concentrations
- memory T cells form cytotoxic (killer) T cells in greater numbers and more quickly, which bind with and destroy more infected cells

Some pathogens, such as the virus that causes influenza ('flu'), mutate regularly, changing the antigens on their surfaces. Memory cells produced as a result of infection by the virus prior to the mutation will be ineffective against the virus after it has mutated. This is because the new antigens are not complementary to the receptors on the memory cells.

Vaccination is a way of stimulating the production of memory cells without exposure to the disease-causing organism.

Key facts you must know and understand

The humoral response

When bacteria enter the body:

- some are ingested by macrophages that then display antigens from the bacteria on their own surface
- some are recognised by inactive B cells with complementary antibodies on their surfaces; the antibodies bind with the antigens of the bacteria

A type of T cell, called a **helper T cell**, binds with the above macrophage and releases chemicals called **interleukins**. These activate the B cells, which divide by mitosis. As they divide, they differentiate into two types of cell:

- **plasma cells** — these are larger than the original B cells and secrete antibodies into the bloodstream
- **memory cells** — these do not release antibodies but remain in the bloodstream for long periods of time and mount a secondary immune response if the same bacterium re-infects the body

Antibodies bring about the destruction of foreign antigens in a number of ways, including:

- agglutination — causing bacteria to form 'clumps' which are then more easily destroyed by white blood cells
- inactivation — neutralising bacterial toxins
- facilitating phagocytosis
- stimulating special proteins (**complement proteins**) to cause lysis (bursting) of bacterial cells

The cell-mediated response

- Viruses entering the body are ingested by macrophages; the viral antigens are displayed on the surface of the macrophages.
- The viruses infect body cells, which also display viral antigens on their surfaces.
- Helper T cells bind with the antigens on the macrophages and secrete interleukins.
- The interleukins activate other T cells that have the appropriate receptors on their surfaces.
- These then divide by mitosis and differentiate into killer T cells and memory T cells.
- The killer T cells bind with the viral antigens on the surfaces of infected cells and secrete **perforins** that destroy the infected cells.

Figure 53 summarises the interaction of the humoral and cell-mediated responses.

examiner tip
Examiners will not reward you for writing about antibodies 'fighting' a pathogen. Use appropriate scientific terminology, such as antibodies cause agglutination or lysis.

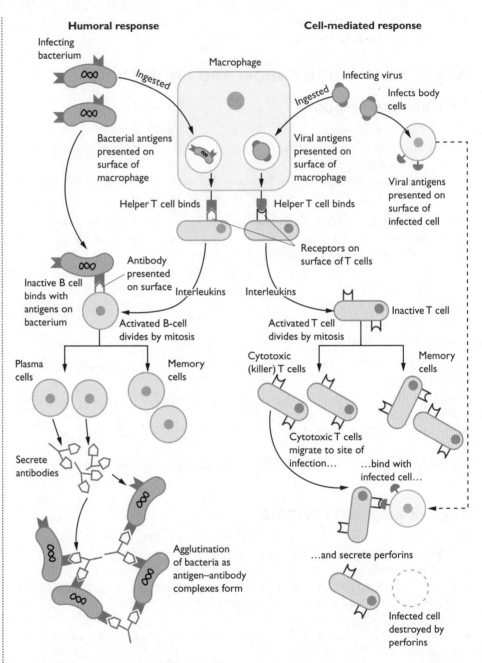

Figure 53 The interaction of the humoral and cell-mediated immune responses

Vaccines and vaccination

A person is exposed to the antigen(s) of a disease-causing organism (causing an immune response) by injecting one of the following:

- an attenuated (weakened) strain of the microorganism (e.g. poliomyelitis, TB and measles vaccines)
- dead microorganisms (e.g. whooping cough and typhoid fever vaccines)
- modified toxins of the causative bacteria (e.g. tetanus and diphtheria vaccines)

examiner tip

The process of producing more active T cells or B cells by mitosis is called **clonal expansion**. A clone is a group of genetically identical cells or individuals.

AQA AS Biology

- isolated antigens (e.g. some influenza vaccines)
- harmless bacteria or yeasts, genetically engineered to carry the antigens of pathogenic microorganisms (e.g. hepatitis B vaccine)

After studying this topic, you should be able to:
- describe the role of lysosomes in the destruction of ingested pathogens
- define the terms antigen and antibody
- explain how the structure of an antibody allows it to form a specific antibody–antigen complex
- describe the differences between humoral and cell-mediated immunity
- describe the term vaccination and explain the difficulty presented by antigenic variability in the production of suitable antigens

Summary

Monoclonal antibodies

Key concepts you must understand

Microorganisms have more than one type of antigen on their surfaces. As a result, more than one type of B cell is stimulated and cloned. The mix of B cells produced is therefore polyclonal and the antibodies are **polyclonal antibodies**.

Monoclonal antibodies are produced from just one type of B cell in response to a single antigen. This means that their action is more specific because they target only that antigen.

Key facts you must know and understand

The high specificity of monoclonal antibodies has attracted the attention of researchers trying to find ways of targeting (for example) cancer cells to kill them with toxic drugs, without affecting any other cells. The principles behind this are:
- produce an antibody that will bind with an antigen found only on the cancer cells
- couple a cytotoxic agent (e.g. a radioactive substance) to the antibody
- inject the antibody/cytotoxin complex into the patient and allow it to target the cancer cells and kill them

Although a strongly radioactive substance is needed, the relatively small amounts required would ensure an effective procedure with few side-effects.

However, there are problems with the procedure. Unless the monoclonal antibody is a human protein, the human immune system will recognise the 'foreign' protein and produce an immune reaction to destroy it. Much research is currently underway to 'humanise' monoclonal antibodies to prevent their rejection by the body.

Knowledge check 33

To make large volumes of monoclonal antibody, scientists fuse a B cell with a tumour cell, to form a new cell called a hybridoma. Explain why (a) a hybridoma will produce large volumes of monoclonal antibody and (b) success is most likely if scientists use a B cell from the person to be injected.

After studying this topic, you should be able to:
- explain what is meant by a monoclonal antibody
- explain how monoclonal antibodies can be used to target harmful cells or specific substances
- evaluate given methodology, evidence and data relating to the use of vaccines and monoclonal antibodies
- develop an understanding of the ethical issues relating to the use of vaccines and monoclonal antibodies

Summary

Questions & Answers

This section contains questions similar in style to those you can expect to see in BIOL1. The limited number of questions in this guide means that it is impossible to cover all the topics and all the question styles, but they should give you a flavour of what to expect. The responses that are shown are real students' answers to the questions.

There are several ways of using this section. You could:
- 'hide' the answers to each question and try the question yourself. It needn't be a memory test — use your notes to see if you can actually make all the points you ought to make
- check your answers against the students' responses and make an estimate of the likely standard of your response to each question
- check your answers against the examiner's comments to see where you might have failed to gain marks
- check your answers against the terms used in the question — for example, did you *explain* when you were asked to, or did you merely *describe*?

Examiner's comments

Each question is followed by a brief analysis of what to watch out for when answering the question (shown by the icon ⓔ). All student responses are then followed by examiner's comments. These are preceded by the icon ⓔ and indicate where credit is due. In the weaker answers, they also point out areas for improvement, specific problems, and common errors such as lack of clarity, weak or non-existent development, irrelevance, misinterpretation of the question and mistaken meanings of terms.

Tips for answering questions

Use the mark allocation. Generally, one mark is allocated for one fact, concept or item in an explanation. Make sure your answer reflects the number of marks available.

Respond appropriately to the command words in each question, i.e. the verb the examiner uses. The terms most commonly used are explained below.
- **Describe** — this means 'tell me about...' or, sometimes, 'turn the pattern shown in the diagram/graph/table into words'; you should not give an explanation.
- **Explain** — give biological reasons for *why* or *how* something is happening.
- **Calculate** — add, subtract, multiply, divide (do some kind of sum!) and show how you got your answer — *always* show your working!
- **Compare** — give similarities *and* differences between...
- **Complete** — add to a diagram, graph, flowchart or table.
- **Name** — give the name of a structure/molecule/organism etc.
- **Suggest** — give a plausible biological explanation for something; this term is often used when testing understanding of concepts in an unfamiliar context.
- **Use** — you must find and include in your answer relevant information from the passage/diagram/graph/table or other form of data.

Question 1 **Heart disease and risk factors**

The diagram shows an external view of the heart.

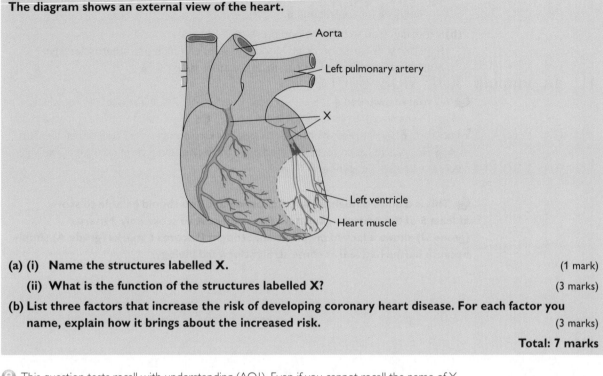

Aorta

Left pulmonary artery

X

Left ventricle

Heart muscle

(a) (i) Name the structures labelled X.   (1 mark)

(ii) What is the function of the structures labelled X?   (3 marks)

(b) List three factors that increase the risk of developing coronary heart disease. For each factor you name, explain how it brings about the increased risk.   (3 marks)

Total: 7 marks

ⓔ This question tests recall with understanding (AO1). Even if you cannot recall the name of X in (a)(i), it is still possible to gain 3 marks by describing its function in (a)(ii). Part (b) clearly requires you to identify a risk factor *and* explain how it increases the risk for each single mark.

(a) (i) X is the cardiac artery **a**.

(ii) The cardiac arteries carry blood to the heart **b** so that it can have oxygen.

(b) Smoking increases cholesterol **c** levels, as can your genes **d**. If you eat too much fatty food you will have high cholesterol levels **e**.

ⓔ **2/7 marks awarded a** The student has not recalled the name and fails to gain an easy mark. **b** It is important to write that these arteries carry blood to heart *muscle*. **c** This is wrong — smoking is not directly linked to high cholesterol levels. **d,e** These factors and their explanations are correct and score 2 marks.

Student B

(a)(i) Coronary artery **a**

(ii) They carry blood rich in oxygen to the cardiac muscle **b** so that it can release energy **c** for contraction **d**.

(b) Stress can lead to higher blood pressure.
Hypertension (sustained high blood pressure) can increase atherosclerosis.
A diet high in saturated fat can increase atherosclerosis **e**.

ⓔ **6/7 marks awarded a** This answer gains 1 mark. Note that this student has not wasted time writing 'The name of the structure labelled X is the…'. **b,d** These statements are correct and gain 1 mark each. **c** Naming respiration as the process releasing energy would have earned the third mark. **e** The student has correctly identified three risk factors and gone on to explain clearly the nature of each risk, thus gaining all 3 marks.

ⓔ **This is a quite straightforward question and you should be able to score at least 5 of the 7 marks allocated. For student A to score only 2 marks (grade U) shows a lack of preparation. Student B scores 6 marks (grade A) simply because he/she had learnt some straightforward biology.**

Question 2 The molecules in our food

A teacher prepared four solutions; one containing glucose, one containing starch, one containing amylase (a starch-digesting enzyme) and one containing sucrose. She labelled them as solutions A, B, C and D. A student carried out the following tests to identify these solutions.

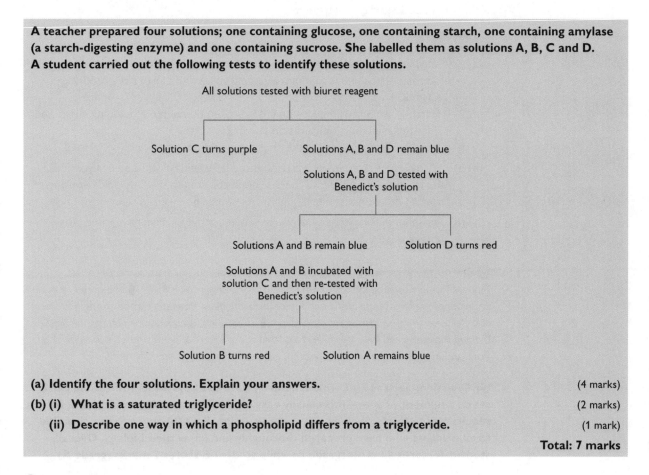

All solutions tested with biuret reagent

Solution C turns purple

Solutions A, B and D remain blue

Solutions A, B and D tested with Benedict's solution

Solutions A and B remain blue

Solution D turns red

Solutions A and B incubated with solution C and then re-tested with Benedict's solution

Solution B turns red

Solution A remains blue

(a) Identify the four solutions. Explain your answers. (4 marks)

(b) (i) What is a saturated triglyceride? (2 marks)

(ii) Describe one way in which a phospholipid differs from a triglyceride. (1 mark)

Total: 7 marks

ⓔ Part (a) requires some thought — you might not have seen information presented in this way before. Part (b) tests recall in a conventional way; in an examination you might prefer to start with this part of the question.

(a) A — starch — identifiable by reaction with iodine/potassium iodide **a**
   B — sucrose — is a non-reducing sugar **b**
   C — amylase — is a protein **c**
   D — glucose — is a reducing sugar **c**

(b) (i) The fatty acids contained in this triglyceride contain no double bonds **d** and tend to be solid around 20°C, and so is a fat and is mainly found in animals.

(ii) A phospholipid contains a phosphate group whereas a triglyceride doesn't **e**.

ⓔ **4/7 marks awarded a** Iodine/potassium iodide is not even mentioned in the question; the student has invented this. **b** The student did not appreciate that amylase only acts on starch and the substance that is changed by this incubation must be starch. **c** These answers are correct and score 2 marks. **d** The student scores I mark for stating there are no double bonds in saturated

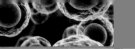

fatty acids but omits to mention that the bonds are between carbon atoms. The rest of the information in this answer is irrelevant and wastes time. **e** The student has made one comparison of the two molecules and gains the mark.

Student B

(a) C — amylase — positive result for protein test and enzymes are proteins **a**

D — glucose — positive result for a reducing sugar and glucose is a reducing sugar **a**

B — starch — when incubated with C it is broken down into a reducing sugar and C is amylase which only acts on starch **a**

A — must be sucrose — not a reducing sugar and not acted on by amylase **a**

(b) (i) Triglycerides contain glycerol and three fatty acids. Saturated triglycerides are triglycerides where all the C–C bonds present in the fatty acids are single bonds and the molecule is fully hydrogenated **b**.

(ii) Phospholipids have two fatty acids whereas triglycerides have three fatty acids **c**.

ⓔ 7/7 marks awarded a This student has identified all four solutions correctly and has supplied logical reasoning to back up the identification, so gains all 4 marks. **b** The presence of only single bonds is addressed, as is the position of these bonds — between carbon atoms in the fatty acid chains — so the student gains both marks. **c** The student has made one comparison between the two molecules and gains the mark. Note that this student's answer gives a different difference from student A. This often happens when a question asks for only one difference.

ⓔ Questions such as 2(a), which require you to use keys for identification, can be set on a number of areas. It is usually easy to obtain some of the marks, but others require you to think carefully about the situation. Part (b) ought to be accessible to all students who have prepared thoroughly and know their biology. Overall, student A scores 4 marks (grade E) while student B scores 7 marks (grade A).

Question 3 The structure and functioning of the digestive system

Figure I shows the main parts of the human digestive system.

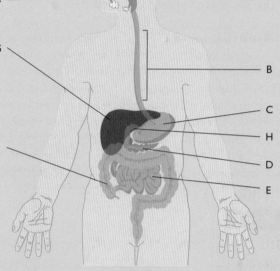

Figure 1

(a) (i) Name the structures labelled **B, C** and **H**. (3 marks)

(ii) Give the letter of the structure that reabsorbs water secreted during digestion. (1 mark)

(b) Figure 2 shows how, during digestion, a molecule of maltose is converted into two molecules of α-glucose.

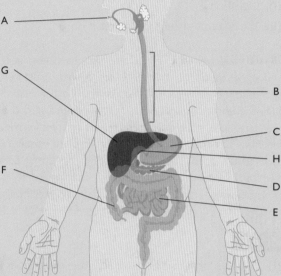

Figure 2

(i) Name the process taking place. (1 mark)

(ii) Explain the role of the enzyme maltase in this reaction. (3 marks)

Total: 8 marks

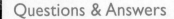
ℯ Part (a)(i) tests your recall of names whereas (a)(ii) asks you to show understanding of function; you might be able to use a letter from the diagram even if you have forgotten the name of the structure. Examiners expect the name of a specific chemical reaction in (b)(i) and for you to show your understanding of *how* enzymes work for the 3 marks in (b)(ii).

Student A

(a)(i) Oesophagus, stomach and small intestine **a**

   (ii) E **b**

(b)(i) Digestion **c**

   (ii) The enzyme speeds up the reaction. **d**

ℯ **3/8 marks awarded a** This student might have been lucky but scores all 3 marks. The answer does not specify which letter relates to which structure, but the sequence of the answers corresponds to the sequence B, C and H in the question. Had the correct answers been given in another sequence, full marks would not have been awarded. **b** The student might have suggested E because, in the diagram, it appears different from H, which s/he identified as the small intestine. Make sure that you know the position of the various regions of the gut. **c** The student has answered as if digestion is a single process, rather than a combination of several processes. The chemical breakdown of food molecules occurs by hydrolysis. The diagram clearly shows the involvement of water in the process as a further clue. **d** Although this student has stated that the enzyme speeds up the reaction, s/he has not given the explanation asked for and gains no mark.

Student B

(a)(i) B — oesophagus; C — stomach; H — duodenum **a**

   (ii) F **b**

(b)(i) Hydrolysis **c**

   (ii) The enzyme acts as a catalyst in the reaction, speeding it up **d**.

ℯ **6/8 marks awarded a** The student has clearly identified the correct structures and gains 3 marks. S/he has identified H as the duodenum; this is not a specification term but is correct (small intestine is the specification term). This is an example of how an answer that is better than the lowest acceptable answer gains a mark. **b** The student is correct and gains this mark. **c** Again, this student scores the mark. **d** The student scores 1 mark for stating that the enzyme is a catalyst. Like student A, however, this student has not explained the role of the enzyme. There are 3 marks allocated to this section of the question and so you should be aware that a simple statement such as 'acts as a catalyst' is not going to score full marks. To score the remaining marks, the students should have gone on to explain how catalysts work — lowering the activation energy by forming an enzyme–substrate complex.

ℯ **This is another quite straightforward question. The first 5 marks should be attainable by any student who has prepared thoroughly. Section (b)(ii) requires you to read the question carefully. Student A scores only 3 marks (grade E) while student B scores 6 marks (grade A).**

Question 4 **The nature and action of enzymes**

The rate of an enzyme-controlled reaction depends on a number of factors, including the concentration of the substrate. Figure 1 shows the rate of reaction of an enzyme-controlled reaction at 25°C at different substrate concentrations.

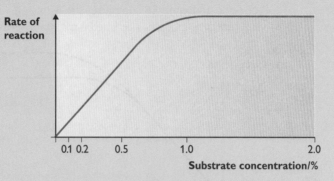

Figure 1

(a) (i) Explain the shape of the graph in terms of kinetic theory and enzyme–substrate complex formation:
A — from substrate concentration of 0.1% to 0.5%
B — from substrate concentration of 1.0% to 2.0% (4 marks)

(ii) Sketch on the graph the curve you would expect if the experiment had been carried out at 35°C rather than 25°C. (1 mark)

(b) Figure 2 represents an energy level diagram of a reaction proceeding without an enzyme, and the same reaction with an enzyme.

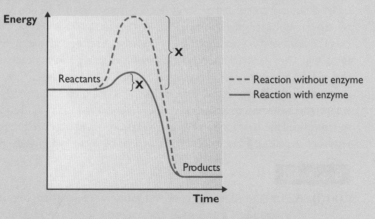

Figure 2

(i) Describe two ways in which the energetics of the two reactions are similar. (1 mark)

(ii) Explain the differences between the regions marked **X** on the diagram. (1 mark)

Total: 7 marks

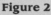 Notice in (a)(i) that you are asked to explain (not describe) and that you are asked to explain in terms of kinetic theory; examiners could not be clearer about what they want in the answer.

Part (b)(i) asks you to describe differences — to turn the differences shown in the curves into words — while (b)(ii) asks for an explanation — reasons for the differences.

Student A

(a) (i) A — the rate of reaction slowly increases from 0.1% to 0.5% because as the substrate concentration increases there are more collisions with the enzyme and more ES complexes are formed **a**.

B — the rate of reaction has reached a maximum between 1.0% and 2.0% **b**.

(ii)

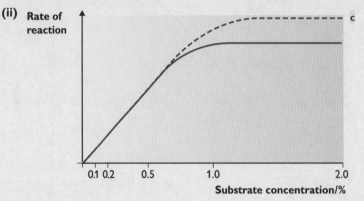

(b) (i) Energy was released from both reactions. Same reactants occur in both reactions **d**.

(ii) With an enzyme, X is smaller than without an enzyme. Enzymes lower activation energy **e**.

ⓔ 3/7 marks awarded a Student A explains clearly how an increase in substrate concentration brings about an increase in the rate of reaction from 0.1% to 0.5% and gains 2 marks. **b** S/he does not explain adequately the shape of the curve between 1.0% and 2.0%. The key feature of the curve here is that it is a horizontal line — meaning no change in rate of reaction. It is not enough to say that it hits a maximum somewhere in that region. **c** The student did not seem to appreciate that at 35°C molecules move about more so the initial rate of reaction would be faster, and scores no marks. **d** Although s/he has included two features from the diagram, only one of them is concerned with energetics and so, as there is only 1 mark for the two ideas, the student fails to score. Read the question carefully and make sure your answer relates precisely to what the examiner has asked. **e** The student has answered correctly and gains the mark.

Student B

(a) (i) A — as the substrate concentration increases there are more active sites available **a** and so at any one time more binding takes place and the reaction rate increases.

B — V-max has occurred because all the active sites available are used at any one time and saturation occurs so the rate of reaction cannot increase any further and stays constant **b**.

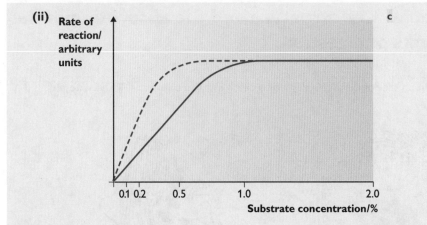

(b)(i) Both the reactants and the products are at the same energy levels in each reaction **d**.

(ii) The activation energy with the enzyme is less than the activation energy without the enzyme **e**.

ⓔ **5/7 marks awarded a** The student has tried to supply extra detail, but gets confused and seems to imply that active sites are part of the substrate molecules, rather than part of the enzyme molecules. S/he scores no marks for this answer. **b** The student gives reasons for the shape of the curve, which is what is needed in an explanation, and gains 2 marks. **c** The student shows that increasing temperature will increase the rate of reaction at low substrate concentrations so that the enzyme will reach its maximum turnover rate at a lower substrate concentration and gains the available 1 mark. **d** The student has clearly identified two features of the energy level diagram that are the same in the two reactions and gains the mark. **e** The student clearly understands this basic concept in enzyme kinetics and gains the mark.

ⓔ **Student A scores a total of 3 marks (grade E); student B scores 5 marks (grade B).**

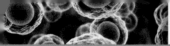

Question 5 Cell structure and the absorption of the products of digestion (I)

The diagram below is drawn from an electron micrograph of a cell from the pancreas. The zymogen granules contain inactive enzymes.

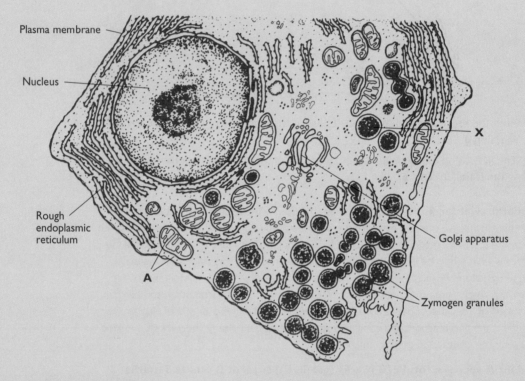

(a) **Name the structures labelled A.** (1 mark)

(b) **Give two pieces of evidence from the diagram that suggest that the cell is synthesising large amounts of protein. Explain your answers.** (4 marks)

(c) **Measure the diameter, in millimetres, of the zymogen granule marked X. The actual diameter of this zymogen granule is 1 μm. Calculate the magnification of this electron micrograph.** (2 marks)

(d) **Explain why the internal membranes of a cell cannot be seen using an optical microscope.** (1 mark)

Total: 8 marks

ⓔ This question tests a number of skills — in an examination you might chose to answer some parts and return to attempt the others, for example part (c), later when your confidence has grown. Notice that the examiners have had to explain about zymogen granules because this is not in the specification. In (b) you need to think about where proteins are made and what then happens to them before you try to interpret the diagram. Be careful about your wording when answering (d).

Student A

(a) Mitochondria **a**

(b) There are a lot of ribosomes present in the cell and these make proteins **b**. The nucleus has many light patches, which indicate that it is coding for much mRNA **c**.

(c) Diameter = 0.7 cm = 700 µm
Magnification = 700 **d**

(d) An optical microscope cannot magnify as highly as an electron microscope **e** and so small objects such as membranes cannot be seen clearly.

ⓔ **3/8 marks awarded a** Like most biology students, this one recognises the mitochondria and gains the mark. **b** Although there are no ribosomes labelled, they are visible on the rough endoplasmic reticulum and do synthesise proteins, so 2 marks are awarded. **c** There is no indication whatsoever that mRNA is being made. **d** The student has measured in centimetres, not millimetres. Neither mark is awarded because the answer is wrong and no method of working is shown. If a correct method had been shown, 1 mark could have been awarded even though the answer is wrong. **e** This student has made a common error and referred to magnification instead of resolution.

Student B

(a) Mitochondria **a**

(b) There is a lot of rough endoplasmic reticulum present and this is concerned with the synthesis of proteins **b**. Second, the large amount of zymogen granules containing inactive enzymes suggests that the enzymes, which are proteins, have been made in the cell **c**.

(c) Magnification = $\dfrac{\text{measured size}}{\text{actual size}}$

Measured = 7 mm = 7000 µm
Actual = 1 µm
Magnification = 7000/1 = 7000 **d**

(d) A light microscope has low resolution **e** and cannot distinguish between the membranes within a cell.

ⓔ **8/8 marks awarded a** This is correct. **b** The student has given one piece of evidence from the diagram and provided an explanation, gaining the first 2 marks. **c** The student uses evidence from the diagram in her/his explanation, gaining a further 2 marks. **d** The student has given the correct answer for 2 marks. S/he has also shown the working: it is easy to get the answer wrong under the stress of an examination but you will usually gain some credit if you show a correct method. **e** The student has correctly identified the low resolution of an optical microscope and gains the mark. Examiners allow 'light microscope' as an alternative to 'optical microscope'.

ⓔ **Student A scores 3 marks (grade E/U), whereas student B scores 8 marks (grade A).**

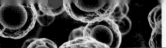
Question 6 Cell structure and the absorption of the products of digestion (II)

Eukaryotic cells are surrounded by a membrane called the plasma membrane. The structure of this membrane is represented by the fluid mosaic model. Substances which enter or leave such a cell must do so through the plasma membrane. Figure 1 represents the fluid mosaic model of membrane structure.

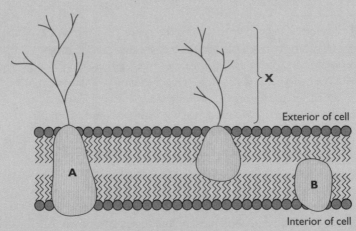

Figure 1

(a) (i)   What is the chemical nature of X? Suggest one possible function of this molecule. (2 marks)

   (ii) Which protein molecule, A or B, could form an ion channel? Explain your answer. (2 marks)

   (iii) Indicate precisely on the diagram one region of this membrane that is hydrophobic. (1 mark)

(b) In an investigation into the permeability of membranes, a student carried out an investigation using discs of beetroot. Beetroot cells contain a purple-red pigment that does not, ordinarily, pass through the plasma membrane. In the investigation, the student:

   (1) cut 10 discs of beetroot

   (2) washed the discs in distilled water until no more colour escaped

   (3) put the washed discs in 10 cm³ distilled water in a test tube taken from a water bath at 20°C

   (4) replaced the test tube in the water bath for 10 minutes

   (5) waited 10 minutes and then measured the coloration of the liquid in the test tube using a colorimeter set to read absorbance

The student repeated this procedure at other temperatures. The results are summarised in Figure 2.

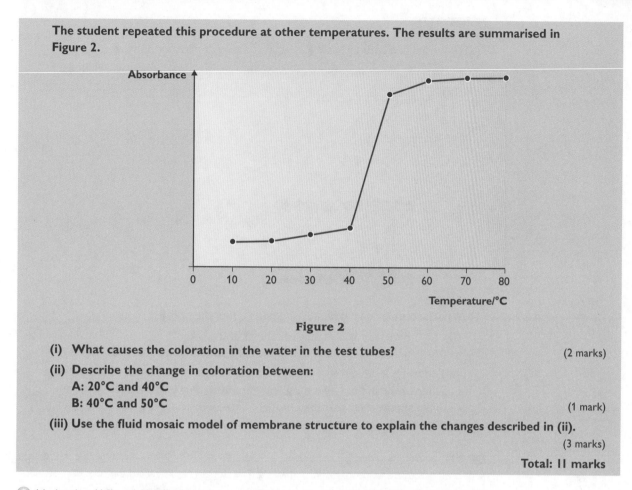

Figure 2

(i)   **What causes the coloration in the water in the test tubes?**   (2 marks)

(ii) **Describe the change in coloration between:**
      A: 20°C and 40°C
      B: 40°C and 50°C   (1 mark)

(iii) **Use the fluid mosaic model of membrane structure to explain the changes described in (ii).**
                                                                                                        (3 marks)

Total: 11 marks

ⓔ Notice that (a)(i) and (ii) offer 2 marks — one for the correct naming/identification and one for an explanation. Be careful in (a)(iii) — the question uses the word 'precisely' so you must be accurate. Part (b) involves an investigation you might have done in class. Notice that (b)(ii) prompts you to 'describe' but (b)(iii) asks you to 'explain' *and* to use your understanding of the fluid mosaic model in your explanation.

Student A

(a)(i) Branched carbohydrate **a** — acts as a receptor for hormones **b**.

(ii) A — because the protein goes past the second layer of phospholipids **c**.

(iii)

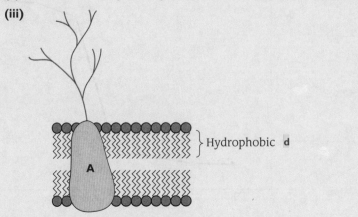

} Hydrophobic **d**

(b)(i) The purple-red pigment as it passes out of the cells **e**.

(ii) A — there is only a slight coloration **f** of the liquid.
B — there is a big difference in the coloration of the liquid from 40°C to 50°C.

(iii) Between 20°C and 40°C, the phospholipid bilayer and proteins in the cell membrane are not affected **g**, but after 40°C they begin to vibrate more, causing the membrane structure to become less stable **h** and therefore letting the purple-red pigment escape.

ⓔ **6/11 marks awarded a** The student has correctly identified X as a carbohydrate, and **b** has suggested a plausible function, gaining 2 marks. **c** The student has identified the correct protein for 1 mark. S/he has not explained clearly the reason for the choice and so does not gain the second available mark. **d** The bracket used by the student just extends into the region of the hydrophilic heads and could be judged to include part of the proteins molecule as well. An examiner would accept this answer, though, and award the 1 mark. **e** The student has gained 1 mark for stating that the pigment passes out of the cells but, not having named diffusion as the process involved, does not gain the second mark. **f** Does this mean there is a slight increase from 20°C to 40°C or does it mean that there is the same small amount present? As a result of this loose wording, the student is not given the mark. **g** The student probably didn't identify the small increase that occurred between 20°C and 40°C and so failed to explain the slight increase in absorbance here. **h** S/he gains 1 mark for identifying the effect of temperature on the membrane.

Student B

(a)(i) X is a carbohydrate and is used for cell recognition **a**.

(ii) A because it is an intrinsic protein (it goes right through the membrane). It provides a hydrophilic pore through the centre of the molecule. **b**

(iii)

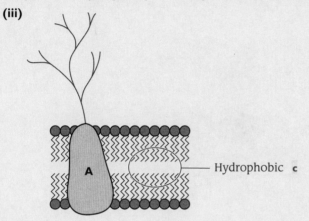

Hydrophobic **c**

(b)(i) Anthocyanin causes the coloration of the water as it diffuses out of the beetroot cells **d**.

(ii) A — there is a slight increase in the coloration.
B — there is a big increase in the coloration. **e**

(iii) Between 20°C and 40°C there is a slight change because as the temperature increases, the molecules in the membrane gain more kinetic energy and so they move around more, which increases the gaps in the membrane and so pigment can diffuse through. **f** After 40°C, the increase in temperature starts to denature some of the proteins in the layer, which means there is a rapid increase in the amount of space for anthocyanin to move through. **g**

ⓔ **10/11 marks awarded a** The student has identified that X is a carbohydrate and suggested a plausible function, so scores 2 marks. **b** The student has identified the correct protein and earns 1 mark. S/he then explains clearly why this protein is chosen and scores the second mark. **c** This addition to the diagram is clear and includes only the hydrophobic fatty acid tails, gaining 1 mark. **d** Examiners would not expect the name of the pigment. This aside, it is clear that this student understands what happens, for both marks. **e** These are unambiguous descriptions for 1 mark. **f** The student has identified and clearly explained the reason for the small increase between 20°C and 40°C and **g** explains the denaturation of proteins above 40°C, gaining 2 marks.

ⓔ **Most students can identify structures in plasma membranes and describe their functions — so make sure that you can. The experiment described in (b) is a fairly standard one. Most students will carry it out for themselves and will be aware of the consequences of heat on plasma membranes. But even if you have not carried it out, you should be able to use your biological knowledge of proteins and lipids to explain these results in terms of altered permeability of the plasma membrane. Student A scores 6 marks (grade C/D); student B scores 10 (grade A).**

Question 7 The lungs, breathing and gas exchange

The diagram shows the structure of the human gas exchange system.

(a) (i)   Name the structures labelled A and B.   (1 mark)

   (ii) What causes air to move into the lungs as the ribs are lifted upwards and outwards and the diaphragm contracts?   (1 mark)

(b) Describe two changes that occur in an asthma attack and explain how these changes affect lung function.   (4 marks)

(c) The substances contained in reliever inhalers are called 'bronchodilators'. Explain why they are given this name.   (2 marks)

Total: 8 marks

ⓔ In (a)(ii), resist the temptation to write six lines about inhalation — the tariff is 1 mark. Part (b) offers 1 mark for each change and 1 mark for the associated explanation. In (c), avoid explaining that a dilator causes dilation — this is not part of the explanation you need to give.

Student A

(a) (i) A — trachea; B — bronchus **a**

   (ii) Air moves in due to the pressure changes. The thorax volume increases, so the pressure in the thorax is less than the atmospheric pressure **b**, so air moves into the lungs until the pressure is equalised.

(b) The bronchioles get narrower **c**, so less air can pass into the lungs **c**. More mucus collects in the bronchioles.

(c) They dilate **d** the bronchus **e**.

ⓔ **3/8 marks awarded a** No mark is awarded — bronchiole was the required name. **b** The student gains the mark but has written far more than was needed. **c** The student understands what happens, but does not explain why the bronchioles get narrower and so gains 2 of the 4 available marks. **d** The word 'dilation' needs to be explained. **e** The student has identified widening of a single bronchus rather than the bronchioles.

Student B

(a) (i) A — trachea; B — bronchiole a

    (ii) The volume of the thorax is increased and therefore the pressure decreases to less than atmospheric pressure, b so air enters the lung and inflates the alveoli until pressure is equal to the atmospheric pressure.

(b) The muscle around the airways contracts c, narrowing the bronchi and bronchioles c. More mucus is also secreted into the airways.

(c) They dilate the bronchioles by making the muscle relax. d

ⓔ 6/8 marks awarded a These answers are correct and gain the mark. b The student scores the 1 mark available here but, like student A, has written far more than was necessary, wasting valuable exam time. c S/he has made two good points but has not related narrowing of the bronchioles with restriction of air movement, thus failing to gain the final marking points. d The student gains 2 marks for identifying the bronchioles and explaining 'dilation'.

ⓔ **Student A scores 3 marks (grade E) while student B scores 6 marks (grade A). Student A failed to gain marks in this question largely through omitting detail. Try to match the detail of your answers to the marks allocated.**

Question 8 The structure and functioning of the heart

The graph shows the pressure changes in the left atrium, left ventricle and aorta during one cardiac cycle.

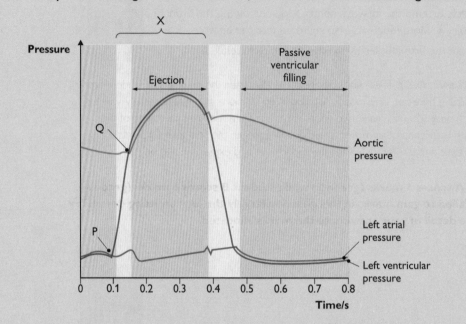

(a) Name the period of the cardiac cycle labelled **X**. Give reasons from the graph for your choice. (2 marks)

(b) What happens at the points in the cycle labelled:

(i) P?

(ii) Q?

Explain your answers. (4 marks)

(c) Sketch a curve on the graph that represents the changes in pressure in the right ventricle. (1 mark)

Total: 7 marks

ⓔ When answering (a), look closely at where period X begins. At P and Q, one curve crosses another — to answer (b) correctly, you must work out from the curves what each relative change in blood pressure will do to heart valves. In (c), think carefully about the structure of the left and right ventricles before you sketch your curve.

Student A

(a) The ventricles are contracting **a** because the pressure in them is rising.

(b)(i) At P, the ventricle contracts **b** and the pressure rises.

(ii) At Q, the ventricle isn't contracting as hard and the pressure doesn't rise as much **c**.

(c)

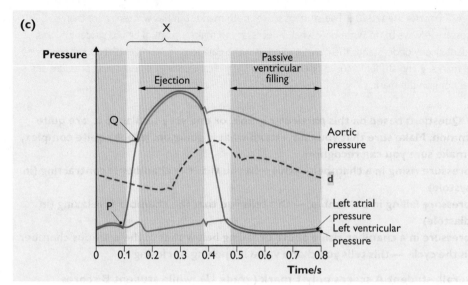

ⓔ 1/7 marks awarded a The student clearly understands what is happening, but has not *named* the process and so scores only 1 mark. Examiners would ignore the reference to both ventricles even though the data concern only the left ventricle. **b** The student has misunderstood the questions and has described what happens between P and Q (rather than at P) and then **c** from Q onwards (rather than at Q) and so scores no marks for (b)(i) or (b)(ii). **d** Although the student's curve shows similar changes at a lower pressure, the changes are out of phase with those of the left ventricle and s/he scores no mark.

Student B

(a) Ventricular systole **a** because the pressure rises, then falls slightly during this period as the left ventricle contracts and ejects blood into the aorta.

(b) (i) At P, the bicuspid valve closes **b** because the pressure in the ventricle rises above the pressure in the atrium.

  (ii) At Q, the aortic valve opens **b** because the pressure in the ventricle gets higher than the pressure in the aorta.

(c)

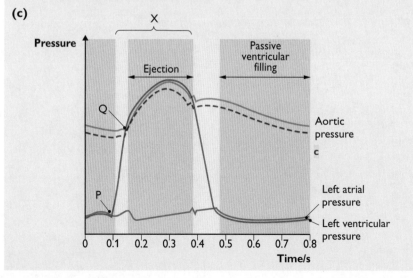

ⓔ **6/7 marks awarded** **a** The student scores both marks, but has written more than is necessary. Always try to write only what is necessary to make a point. **b** Unlike student A, this student clearly understands the question and uses the data to give sound explanations, so scoring all 4 marks. **c** The student's curve does not show a significant enough difference in pressure and so does not gain the mark.

ⓔ **Questions based on this particular graph, or one very similar to it, are quite common. Make sure that you understand what is going on. It looks quite complex, so make sure you can recognise:**

- **pressure rising in a chamber — this tells you that the chamber is contracting (in systole)**
- **pressure falling in a chamber — this tells you that the chamber is relaxing (in diastole)**
- **pressure in a chamber rising above or falling below that of the previous chamber in the cycle — this tells you that a valve is opening or closing**

Overall, student A scores only 1 mark (grade U), while student B scores 6 marks (grade A).

Question 9 Smoking and respiratory disease

In 1951, Dr Richard Doll began a survey into the health of British doctors and their smoking habits. The graphs show the survival rates from age 35 of doctors born at different times.

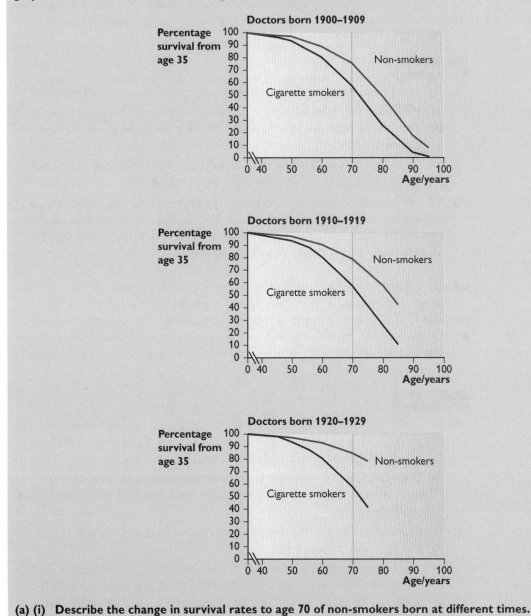

(a) (i) Describe the change in survival rates to age 70 of non-smokers born at different times. (2 marks)

(ii) Suggest a reason for the difference in survival rates that you described in your answer to (i).

(2 marks)

(b) The survival rate to age 70 for the three groups of doctors who smoked is the same. Suggest a reason for this. (3 marks)

(c) The data show a survival rate of 58% for smokers who were born between 1920 and 1929. Explain why this figure may be misleading and how the presentation of the data could be improved. (5 marks)

Total: 12 marks

ⓔ Part (a)(i) involves comparing all three graphs before you answer. Parts (a)(ii) and (b) require you to think of other risk factors. Part (c) is a good test of your ability to examine data and conclude critically (AO3).

Student A

(a) (i) The doctors born later have an even better chance of surviving **a** compared with the non-smokers.

(ii) They have a better chance of living to 70 now because people eat healthier food. **b**

(b) The doctors who smoked would still be affected by the chemicals **c** in the smoke and may have died from heart disease or lung cancer. **d**

(c) It's only an average figure — some people smoke more and some smoke less. **e** So the results aren't necessarily the same for someone who smokes twenty cigarettes a day and someone who smokes only five a day. The graphs should show the results for different amounts of smoking.

ⓔ **4/12 marks awarded a** The student has answered the wrong question and described how the difference between smokers and non-smokers changes. **b** The student appreciates that diet is significant, for 1 mark. **c** The reference to chemicals in the smoke is vague and scores no marks. **d** S/he realises, however, that either heart disease or cancer could be the consequence and scores 1 mark. **e** The student appreciates one limitation of the data and goes on to suggest a reasonable improvement to score 2 marks.

Student B

(a) (i) The doctors born between 1900 and 1909 have a survival rate of 75%. Ten years later the survival rate had increased **a** to 80% **b** and for doctors born between 1920 and 1929, it had reached 85%.

(ii) There has been a general improvement in the standard of living. Diet improved **c**, which meant that people were better able to defend themselves **d** against disease.

(b) The living standards didn't improve enough to compensate for the effects of nicotine **e** in the tobacco smoke.

(c) The result is obviously only an average for all smokers. Heavy and light smokers are included **f** in the one figure. Also, it doesn't differentiate between the time periods **g** over which people smoked. Some may have been smoking for years and others only for months or weeks. Some cigarettes are more dangerous than others because they either don't have filter tips **h** or they have stronger tobacco. **i**

It would be better to show different graphs for different levels of smoking and for different time periods that people have been smoking. **j**

(e) **10/12 marks awarded** **a** The student describes correctly the survival trend in the non-smokers and **b** scores the second point by illustrating the answer with data from the graphs. **c** The student recognises the importance of diet and, although s/he could have expressed it better, **d** goes on to explain why, and so scores 2 marks. **e** The student clearly appreciates that there was an improvement in living conditions during the period of the investigation but that it seems not to have been enough to offset the effects of the toxins in cigarette smoke. S/he incorrectly identifies nicotine as a carcinogen and scores 1 mark. **f–i** The student provides four explanations of how the data can be misleading and in **j** provides a suggestion of how the data can be represented better, so gains all 5 marks.

(e) **This question tests your ability to analyse data that at first sight are a little complex. The key is to first look at the three graphs separately and understand each one, before trying to integrate the data. When analysing data, you often have to deal with means (averages). This can be a strength of the investigation, as more results improve reliability. If the mean hides several uncontrolled variables that could influence the results, then dealing with the mean would be a weakness. You must think carefully about the situation you are dealing with. Overall, student A scores 4 marks (grade E), while student B, who is better able to analyse the data, scores 10 marks (grade A).**

Question 10 Monoclonal antibodies

Several monoclonal antibodies have been developed to help with the treatment of heart disease. One of these targets a gene that controls the metabolism of lipids. The antibody carries a substance that 'knocks out' the gene. Experiments using mice have shown that use of the drug significantly lowers levels of cholesterol in the plasma.

(a) Suggest how monoclonal antibodies are able to target a particular gene precisely. (3 marks)

(b) Suggest how use of the antibody described may reduce the risk of heart disease. (3 marks)

(c) Suggest why the results of this research should be treated with some caution. (2 marks)

(d) Comment on the ethics of this research. (4 marks)

Total: 12 marks

ⓔ Read the second sentence of the question carefully when answering (b). Part (c) is a straightforward test of AO3. Part (d) also tests AO3 — avoid an emotional response and try to present a balanced answer.

Student A

(a) Monoclonal antibodies are only made by one type of cell so they are only active against one specific substance **a**. This antibody just targets one gene.

(b) Cholesterol blocks arteries **b** and can cause heart disease, so by lowering the levels of cholesterol, there is less risk of a heart attack.

(c) Mice are not the same as humans **c** and might respond differently **d**.

(d) It is not fair to research on mice because they can't say no **e** and may suffer. Altering the gene may do more than just affect the cholesterol levels. It might affect 'good cholesterol' **e** in the body.

ⓔ **6/12 marks awarded a** The student explains the concept of specificity (only active against one substance) and gains 1 mark. **b** S/he explains that cholesterol can lead to blocked arteries and scores 1 mark. **c** The student appreciates the problem of using a different species that **d** might not react like humans. **e** The student makes two reasonable points and gains 2 marks. Notice, though, that both are negative — s/he has not tried to present both sides of the issue

Student B

(a) The substance carried by the antibody will have a unique shape **a** and so will be able to bind with only one substance **b**, in this case the gene.

(b) A high cholesterol level is a key risk factor in coronary heart disease **c**. So, by lowering the level of cholesterol, the risk of heart disease is lowered.

(c) Mice are a different species and the results may not be transferable to humans **d** because of different metabolism **d**.

(d) There are always problems in experimenting on animals. Clearly, the animals are not there by choice **e** (as human volunteers in clinical trials would be) and there may be harmful side effects **f** from altering the gene. Lipids are important substances in the body. Altering the lipid metabolism might affect the phospholipids **g** in plasma membranes. On the other hand, it may be worth 'sacrificing' a few mice if the research might lead to saving thousands or even millions of human **h** lives.

🅔 9/12 marks awarded **a** The student has included the importance of shape in explaining **b** the concept of specificity and scores 2 marks. **c** The student has explained the risk of high cholesterol levels in coronary heart disease, but not explained why, so scoring 1 mark. Note that neither student suggested an explanation of the link to targeting the gene that controls lipid metabolism. Make sure that if 3 marks are available, your answer has sufficient detail to gain them. **d** The student gains both marks for explaining the difficulty of interpreting research carried out on different species. **e–g** The student has given three ethical issues. **h** S/he has also tried to put both sides of the argument — the case for and the case against — and scores all 4 marks for a well-balanced answer. If you are asked to comment on the ethics of a piece of research, do not allow yourself to make a purely emotional argument, no matter how much you believe it. Always try to put both sides of the argument.

🅔 **Overall, student A scores 6 marks (grade D) and student B scores 9 marks (grade B). Both students showed a general appreciation of the problems in this question, but student A, once again, was not able to supply sufficient detail.**

Knowledge check answers

1 By damaging the cells of the host and by producing toxins

2 Increase exercise; stop smoking; cut down on alcohol intake

3 **(a)** two molecules of α-glucose, **(b)** one molecule of α-glucose and one molecule of fructose, **(c)** one molecule of α-glucose and one molecule of galactose

4 A molecule of water (H_2O) is eliminated during the condensation reaction.

5 **(a)** glycosidic; **(b)** peptide

6 It has more than one polypeptide/more than one chain of amino acids.

7 Unlike a polysaccharide and a polypeptide, a lipid molecule is not a polymer because it is not formed as a chain of monomers.

8 A starch molecule is too large to cross the wall of the gut. It must be hydrolysed into its component monomers (monosaccharides), which are small enough to cross the gut wall.

9 The active site, which binds with the substrate molecule(s), is part of the tertiary (3D) structure of the enzyme molecule.

10 The shape of the active site is complementary to the shape of only one (or only one type of) substrate molecule.

11 An increase in the number of collisions between enzyme and substrate molecules is opposed by an increase in the number of enzyme molecules that are denatured (undergo a permanent change in shape).

12 You should first realise that having a lower minimum resolution is the same as having a higher resolving power. You should have found from the table that the resolution of an optical microscope is 0.2 μm and that of a TEM is 1 nm. Since there are 10^3 nm in 1 μm, then 0.2 μm = 200 nm and the TEM has a resolving power that is 200 times greater than the optical microscope.

13 The nucleus controls which proteins will be made; ribosomes on the rough endoplasmic reticulum make the proteins; the rough endoplasmic reticulum transports the proteins to the Golgi apparatus; the Golgi apparatus modifies the proteins and releases them in vesicles.

14 **(a)** because it is a patchwork of different molecules — phospholipids, proteins and carbohydrates; **(b)** because the molecules move about laterally.

15 Each is a fatty acid (see Figure 14 to remind yourself).

16 The cell will gain water. Osmosis occurs from a higher (less negative) water potential to a lower (more negative) water potential. In this case, osmosis will occur from the solution, with a water potential of −10 kPa, into the cell, with a water potential of −20 kPa.

17 A transport protein (which is different from the type that transports glucose) carries one amino acid molecule and one sodium ion into the epithelial cell by facilitated diffusion. Sodium ions are actively pumped out of the base of the epithelial cell by active transport; amino acid molecules pass out by facilitated diffusion.

18 Each has a shape that is complementary either to a glucose molecule or to an amino acid molecule.

19 The protein channels in the plasma membranes of gut epithelial cells co-transport both sodium chloride and glucose, so both must be present in the ORT solution.

20 Tidal volume = pulmonary ventilation rate/breathing rate. [Make sure you are confident in changing the subject of an equation.]

21 Ventilating the lungs replenishes oxygen-rich air in the alveoli, increasing the oxygen diffusion gradient into the blood. It also replaces air that has a high carbon dioxide concentration with air that has a low carbon dioxide concentration, increasing the carbon dioxide diffusion gradient out of the blood.

22 Your answer will probably include five of the following: diaphragm muscles contact; diaphragm pulled downwards; (external) intercostal muscles contract; ribs pulled upwards; volume of thorax cavity increases; pressure in thorax cavity decreases; air moves (from atmosphere) into lungs down pressure gradient.

23 **(a)** The cavities have a smaller volume than the alveoli that have been destroyed, so the tidal volume becomes less. **(b)** The surface area of the cavities is smaller than that of the alveoli that have been destroyed.

24 People with an inadequate diet lack energy and/or vital nutrients to maintain a strong immune system. People infected by HIV have an immune system that is already compromised.

25 The solid particles inhaled with coal dust cause scarring of the lung tissue, with resulting loss of elasticity.

26 During diastole, the muscular wall of a heart chamber is relaxing; during systole, it is contracting.

27 Since cardiac output = heart rate × stroke volume, stroke volume = cardiac output/heart rate = 3000 cm^3 per minute/60 beats per minute = 50 cm^3.

28 This valve will close when the pressure in the right ventricle (pushing it shut) is greater than the pressure in the right atrium (pushing it open).

29 One heart beat takes 0.8 seconds, so heart rate = 60/0.8 = 75 beats $minute^{-1}$.

30 **(a)** The delay allows time for the atria to empty before the ventricles contract. **(b)** By contracting from the base upwards, each ventricle squeezes out all the blood. (Think of squeezing a toothpaste tube from the bottom rather than from the middle.)

31 A glycoprotein has carbohydrate chains attached to it (see Figure 31); a protein does not.

32 Memory B cells produce appropriate antibodies very quickly and destroy the bacterium before it can cause harm.

33 **(a)** Like tumour cells, the hybridoma will divide rapidly; like B cells, the progeny cells will produce one type of antibody. **(b)** Antibodies are proteins and can act as antigens. If the B cell is from the person who will be injected with the monoclonal antibodies, the antibodies will not be rejected.

A

α-1,4-glycosidic bond   14
α-glucose   12, 13, 14, 21
α-helix   16
absorption, digestion   20, 32–36
activation energy   22
active site, enzymes   22, 23
active transport   35, 36
agglutination of bacteria   55
allosteric site, enzymes   26
alveoli, gas exchange   39–43
amino acids   15–16
    absorption of   36
amylase   21
aneurysm   52–53
antibodies   53–57
    monoclonal   57, 82–83
antibody–antigen complex   53
antigens   53–54, 55–57
asthma   45–46
atheroma   52
atherosclerosis   52–53
atrioventricular node (AVN)   51

B

β-pleated sheet   16
B lymphocytes (B cells)   54, 55, 56, 57
bacteria   9
    body's response to   55–56
    causing cholera   37–38
    causing pulmonary TB   43–44
biochemical tests   18–19
blood pressure   10, 47
breathing   39–41

C

cancers   10–11
carbohydrates   12–15
cardiac cycle   48–51
cardiac output   48
casual relationships   11
catalysts, enzymes as   22
cell fractionation   30

cell-mediated immune response   54, 55–56
cell structure   30–32
    plasma membranes   32–36
cholera   37–38
cholesterol   10, 34, 82
chromosomes   15
circulatory system   47–48
clonal expansion   56
competitive inhibitors 25–26
complementary shapes, enzymes   22–23
concentration gradient   34–35
condensation reactions   13–14, 16
conformational change, enzymes   26
coronary heart disease (CHD)   9–10, 51–53, 59–60
correlation   8, 11

D

denaturation, enzymes   24–25
diastole   47
diffusion   34–36
    gas exchange in alveoli   39, 42–43
    particles across membrane   34–36
digestive system   20–21, 63–64
dipeptides   15–16
disaccharides   13, 14, 15, 18
double circulation   47

E

emphysema   44–45
endoplasmic reticulum (ER)   31–32
enzyme–substrate complex   22–23
enzymes   22–23
    factors affecting action   23–27
epidemiology   8
epithelial cells   30–32
    plasma membranes   32–36

F

facilitated diffusion   35, 36
fluid-mosaic model   32, 33, 70
fractionation   30
fungi   9

G

gas exchange   39–40, 42–43
α-glucose   12, 13, 14, 21
glycosidic bonds   13, 14–15
Golgi apparatus   31, 32

H

heart
    cardiac cycle   49–51
    disease   9–10, 51–53, 59–60
    structure   47–48, 76–78
heart rate   48
α-helix   16
helper T cells   55
humoral immune response   54, 55, 56
hydrolysis reactions   14, 17, 20, 21
hydrolytic enzymes   20

I

immune response   53–57
immunological memory   54
induced-fit model of enzyme action   23
infectious diseases   8–9
    body's reaction to   53–57
ingestion   20
    of pathogens   55–56
integral proteins   33, 34
intercostal muscles   41
interleukins   55, 56
ion channels   32
ion pores, proteins   34

K

kinetic energy   24, 35, 65

L

lactose intolerance   15
lifestyle and disease   9–10, 43
lipids   17–18
   test for   19
lock-and-key model   22–23
lungs
   breathing   39, 41
   diseases of   10–11, 43–46
   gas exchange   39–40, 42–43
   structure   40
lymphocytes   54
lysis (bursting)   55
lysosomes   31

M

macromolecules   12, 15
macrophages   44, 54, 55
magnification   30
maltase   21
maltose   13, 14, 21, 63
memory cells   54–55
microscopes   27–29
microvilli   32, 36
mitochondria   31
monoclonal antibodies   57, 82–83
monomers, hydrolysis of   20, 21
monosaccharides   12–13
myogenic, heartbeat   48

N

non-competitive inhibitors   26–27
non-reducing sugars, test for   19
nucleus   31, 68

O

optical microscopes   28, 29
optimum temperature   24
organelles   30–31
osmosis   35

P

partial pressure, gases   40
pathogens   8–9, 54

peptide bonds   15–16
perforins   55, 56
peripheral proteins   33–34
pH, effect on enzyme action   24–25
phospholipid bilayer   32–34
phospholipids   17
plasma cells   55
plasma membranes   15
   as a barrier   32–34
   transport processes   34–35
β-pleated sheet   16
polyclonal antibodies   57
polypeptides   15–17
polysaccharides   15
primary immune response   54
primary structure, proteins   16
prokaryotic cells   37
proteins   15–17
   test for   19
pulmonary fibrosis   45
pulmonary tuberculosis   43–44
pulmonary ventilation rate   39
pumps, carrier proteins   35
Purkyne tissue   50, 51

Q

quaternary structure, proteins   17

R

reducing sugars   18, 19
resolution of microscopes   27–28
respiratory disease   10–11, 43–46
ribosomes   31–32
risk factors   8, 9–10, 59–60
rough ER   31–32, 68–69

S

saturated fatty acids   18
scanning electron microscopes   29
secondary immune response   54, 55
secondary structure, proteins   16

β-sheet   16
sinoatrial node (SAN)   51
small intestine   21
   absorption from   32–36
   epithelial cells   30–32
smoking   10–11, 43, 44–45, 79–81
smooth ER   32
starch   15
   digestion of   21
   test for   19
stroke volume   48
substrate concentration, enzymes   25, 26, 27, 65–67
substrates, enzymes   22–23
sucrose   13, 18
sugars, testing for   18, 19
systole   47

T

T lymphocytes (T cells)   54, 55
temperature and enzyme action   24
tertiary structure, proteins   16
tests for biochemicals   18–19
tidal volume   39
transmembrane proteins   33–34
transmission electron microscopes   28, 29
transport proteins   32, 34, 35, 36
triglycerides   17, 18

U

unsaturated fatty acids   18

V

vaccines/vaccination   56–57
ventilation rate   39
viruses   8–9, 54–55

W

water potential   35, 38